"An easy, breezy, and hugely informative read."

David Goldbloom, OC, MD, FRCPC
Professor of Psychiatry, University of Toronto

"Do yourself a favour and read this book. You won't find this crucial information anywhere else."

Paula Brook, Author and former Editor-in-Chief
of *Western Living Magazine*

"How do you even ASK to get help for any problems around your bum? This book gives you the language to ask your questions and provides crystal clear answers that you will not find elsewhere."

Nancy Epstein, MD, FRCSC
Lecturer, Department of Ophthalmology and
Vision Sciences, University of Toronto

"Destined to be the *'number two'* best seller of all time!
Internationally respected Colorectal Surgeon, Marcus Burnstein, shares valuable insights and wisdom in a tremendously informative, easily readable, and entertaining book. A truly valuable resource for health care providers, medical and healthcare students, AND ANYONE WITH AN ANUS. What you need and want to know, and more, about the function and care of your bottom end."

Dr. Kenneth Robb, Associate Professor
of Medicine, University of Toronto

"A 'poop-o-gram'? Who knew? Turns out Dr. Marcus Burnstein does. This is a terrific owner's and user's manual for your keister. Enjoy."

Howard Epstein, LLB, MLA, Nova Scotia (*ret.*)

"I am very impressed with *Bummer*. I especially liked the use of patient examples which makes it more readable and relatable. The more people that read this book the better!"

Catherine Lawrence, LLB

"It's an absolute *tour de force*. So well written. You continue to amaze me Dr. Burnstein!"

Chad Ball, MD, FRCSC
Professor of Surgery, University of Calgary

"What a *Bummer*! A lot goes on down there – more than you can imagine. Now we can all know what goes on and it is told to us in a way that we can easily understand. Clearly written, with one topic leading to the next, *Bummer* delves into the workings of our bottom end. Filled with important health information and humour. Thank you, Dr. Marcus."

Myrna Yazer, BN
Research Manager, Pain Management Unit,
QEII Health Sciences Centre (*ret.*)

"*Bummer* illuminates all the issues that exist 'where the sun don't shine.' In this very informative book, Dr. Marcus Burnstein lays out various anal and colorectal problems in an understandable, easy-to-read fashion that patients (and their physicians!) will benefit from tremendously. One of our favourite sections is Dr. Burnstein's reflections on what it means to be a surgeon and how he tries to pass along that legacy to his trainees. *Bummer* is an important offering from one of Canada's most highly respected colorectal surgeons, and is for all those interested in what goes on with the back passage."

Dr. Ameer Farooq, MD, FRCSC, Associate Professor,
Queen's University and Dr. Chad Ball, MD, FRCSC,
Professor of Surgery, University of Calgary, Hosts of
Cold Steel: The Canadian Journal of Surgery Podcast

"One of the most brilliant minds of all time, Marcus Aurelius, said, 'When you arise in the morning, think of what a privilege it is to be alive, to think, to enjoy, to love.' Another brilliant Marcus gave me the ability to continue to enjoy that privilege. When I needed surgery, my GI specialist recommended I have the operation 'now that we have Marcus Burnstein!' He told me that Dr. Burnstein was one of only a few surgeons in Canada who could do the surgery that I required. So, thank you Marcus! And thank you for *Bummer*. Very easy to read and extremely informative."

Angelo Contardi, President & CEO, Pizzaville Inc.

"Problems 'down there' are common, but questions about anal health can be uncomfortable to ask. *Bummer* asks the important questions and provides clear answers. Dr. Burnstein gets to the bottom of things in an extremely readable, understandable, and entertaining way."

John Tory, Order of Ontario, former Mayor of Toronto

BUMMER

What You Need to Know
About Anal Health

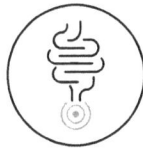

MARCUS BURNSTEIN, MD

COLORECTAL SURGEON

ISBN 978-1-7381093-0-2 (Paperback)
ISBN 978-1-7381093-1-9 (e-Book)

First Printing

Editor: Catherine Leek of Green Onion Publishing
Cover and Interior Design and Layout: Kim Monteforte Book Design & Self-Publishing Services
Illustrator: Mat Brown

To Robin McLeod, OC, MD, FRCSC
My dear friend and colleague

A good reliable set of bowels is worth more to a man [or woman] than any quantity of brains.

Josh Billings, American humourist, 1818-1885

Table of Contents

Foreword

The anus is a part of the body that for most people requires little thought or concern – that is, until it starts to misbehave or go wrong. When this happens, such a small part of the body can cause significant distress and trouble. Symptoms from the bottom area can be problematic and occasionally even very disabling, as well as being embarrassing. They can be short-lived and often caused by common or self-resolving problems, such as haemorrhoids, but occasionally can be due to life-threatening conditions, including cancer.

The art of working out the cause of someone's symptoms so that the science of treating them appropriately can be put into action requires an experienced specialist in this field and, for me, there is none better than Dr. Marcus Burnstein. Having been trained by Marcus whilst learning colorectal surgery at the University of Toronto, his attention to detail in listening to patients, and in picking up subtle clues whilst examining them, are lessons I have taken with me and put into my own clinical practice to this day, along with trying to mirror the kind way that he puts his patients at ease in potentially difficult and embarrassing clinical encounters.

Bummer outlines the range of conditions that can affect this most intimate and private of body areas in a way that is as readable to the non-medically trained person in the street as it is to a qualified colorectal specialist. *Bummer* is informative, interesting, reflective and at times funny – all in appropriate measures – just like its author!

JUSTIN DAVIES
Consultant Colorectal Surgeon and Deputy Medical Director,
Cambridge University Hospitals
President Elect, Association of Coloproctology of Great Britain and Ireland
President, Royal Society of Medicine Section of Coloproctology

Acknowledgements

I have had a lot of moral and editorial support from my children, Eli and Jessica. Eli, a professional writer and editor, provided me with many tweaks that improved the style and clarity of *Bummer*. My original manuscript included graphic photographs that generated Eli's insightful editorial comments, "Yeesh!" and "For the love of God!" I decided to go with a professional illustrator.

Speaking of which, I want to thank Mat Brown whose valuable illustrations tremendously enhance the descriptions of anatomy and operations.

I want to especially thank my editor, Catherine Leek, who guided me through the process with efficiency, expertise, and professionalism. And thanks go to Rae Keen, who put me in touch with Catherine. Catherine brought in Kim Monteforte whose creative designs, from cover to cover, have made *Bummer* look fabulous.

I would never have written a book about anal health if I had not been encouraged to do so by friends and colleagues. I want to particularly acknowledge Nancy Epstein and David Goldbloom who persuaded me that I had something to offer and for their review of the manuscript. Early versions were reviewed by Robert Grant, Elizabeth Currie, Paula Brook, Catherine Lawrence, Ken Robb, Ameer Farooq, Chad Ball, Linda Epstein, Angelo Contardi, Myrna Yazer, Howard Epstein, and John Tory. Thank you for your helpful input.

The University of Toronto Residency Program in Colorectal Surgery has attracted exceptional surgeons from around the world who have gone on to stellar careers. One of our most illustrious alumni is Professor Justin Davies of the University of Cambridge. Justin is currently President of The Association of Coloproctology of Great Britain and Ireland, and President of The Royal Society of Medicine

Section of Coloproctology. He is also a great surgeon. I am very grateful for, and sincerely honoured by, his foreword for *Bummer*.

A special thank you to crime-writer and lawyer, Robert Rotenberg. I told him I was working on a book tentatively entitled *Anus: An Owner's Manual*. He gave me *Bummer*. Better.

The real force behind this enterprise has been my wife, Ruth, who steadily encouraged me to write *Bummer* and has been my primary editor. I am tremendously grateful to her. I really enjoyed the process of bringing *Bummer* to life, and I am proud of the finished product.

Surgery is a craft, not an art. It is much less about talent than it is about training. I have been well trained and am profoundly indebted to the surgeons who trained me. I am also indebted to many colleagues, residents, and students at St. Michael's Hospital who have taught, challenged, and supported me, especially James Waddell, Marisa Louridas, Tyler Chesney, and Nancy Baxter.

During my General Surgery residency at the University of Toronto, my interest in Colorectal Surgery was sparked by Dr. Zane Cohen. Zane was at the forefront of reconstructive operations for rectal cancer and ulcerative colitis. It was exciting to be a resident on Zane's service. I am very grateful for his mentorship, support, and friendship.

While training in Toronto I had the opportunity to work with the late Dr. Earl Myers. Dr. Myers was known as the Rear Admiral. He was superb. I still do many things just the way he showed me.

As a Colorectal Surgery fellow at the Lahey Clinic in Massachusetts, I was the junior member of a surgical family. I had a big brother, David Schoetz, an uncle, John Coller, and a father, the late Malcolm "Mike" Veidenheimer. I was incredibly fortunate to spend every day in the company of these master craftsmen. I especially want to thank David Schoetz, a wonderful surgeon, and a devoted mentor. David has been the most important role model of my career.

I have sought input from colleagues, both surgical and non-surgical. I have sought input from lay people, both with and without anal complaints. The feedback has been positive. A friend texted, "*Bummer* is full of important information for anyone who has an anus." My hope is that patients, as well as people with an interest in gastrointestinal health and disease, will find *Bummer* to be an informative, helpful, and entertaining read.

Out of the Shadows

The tubular gut is a 20-foot subway line that runs from the mouth to the anus. Food enters at one end. Poop comes out at the other. Between the beginning and end of that journey, the gut digests the food, absorbs the nutrients and water, and prepares the rest for evacuation out the anus (see Figure 1).

We're here to talk about that last part.

Figure 1

The Digestive System

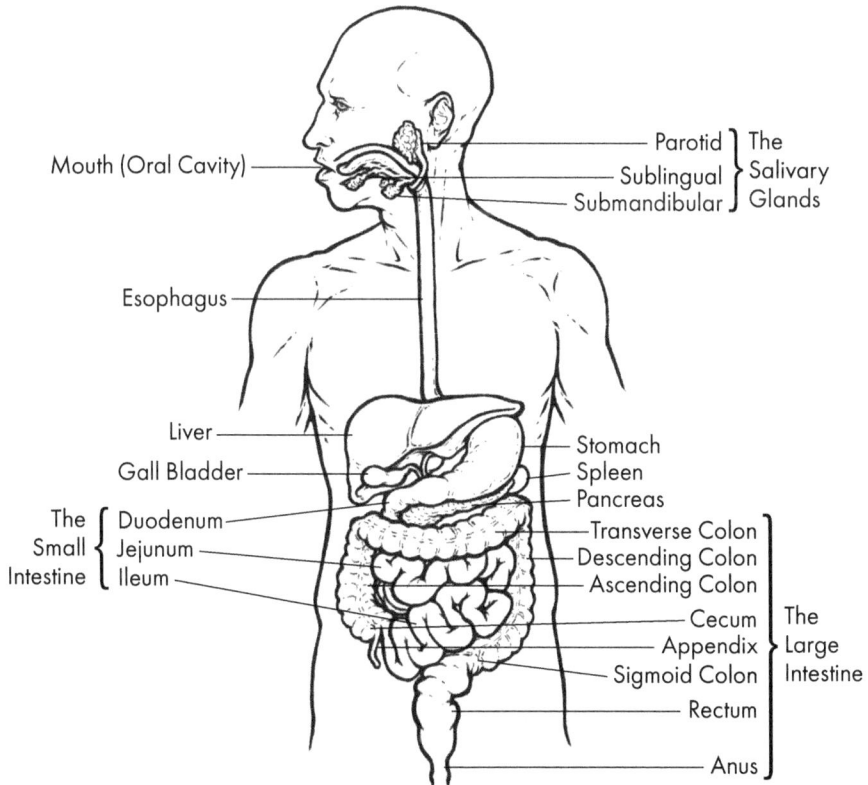

THE BEGINNING AND THE END

The intake phase of digestion can be a spectacular sensory experience. It may be shared with others, savoured enthusiastically, and documented by selfies. The elimination phase, by contrast, is a solitary and rarely memorable mission. Not a lot of selfies.

Despite their obvious differences, the two ends of the gut do have a few things in common: both get a lot of wear and tear, both interact with the outside environment, and both are common sites of disease and dysfunction.

Yet while almost everyone sees a dentist for routine checkups and the maintenance of oral health, regular visits to an anal doctor aren't part of standard healthcare. I am not suggesting they should be. But anal problems are very common, many of them are preventable, and all are manageable, if not curable. Also, anal problems don't get a lot of press. That, in a nutshell, is why I wrote *Bummer*.

In the pages to come, I discuss the common problems that afflict the anus. I look at the way Colorectal Surgeons like me diagnose and treat these problems. And I look at some of the ways we can take better care of our bums in our everyday lives.

WHEN YOU SEE A COLORECTAL SURGEON

Doctors like to have an approach for everything. Algorithms, the rules and steps to solving problems, exist for almost everything in medicine and surgery. As much as possible, doctors try to ensure that their algorithms are guided by data. This is called "evidence-based medicine." Algorithms help us provide good care and avoid errors, especially errors of omission.

Medicine and Surgery

Some patients who come to see me do not fully understand the difference. Most people appreciate that there are Family Doctors (the speciality of Family Medicine, in my opinion) and specialists. There are two types of specialists, medical and surgical, and some parts of the human body engage both types. The gastrointestinal (GI) tract, for example, is looked after by medical specialists called Gastroenterologists, as well as by surgeons, called General Surgeons. Bones and joints are looked after by Rheumatologists and Orthopaedic Surgeons. The heart by Cardiologists and Cardiac Surgeons. Some body parts get only one specialty; the eye and the ear are each looked after by specialists who provide both medical and surgical care to their patients. OB-GYN specialists do the medical, the surgical, and the obstetrical care for their patients. Unlimited sub-specialization within medicine and surgery makes it even more confusing. There are General Surgeons, like me, who only look after the colon, rectum, and anus, and are called Colorectal Surgeons. Some other General Surgeons only look after the liver, pancreas, and bile ducts. The eye is so complicated that there are Ophthalmologists, who only look after the front of the eye, and others who only look after the back of the eye. Orthopaedic operations can be so technically challenging that Orthopaedic Surgery has a sub-specialty for every joint in the human skeleton. Is all this specialization a good thing? Overall, I think it is. There is a lot of evidence that sub-specialization translates into better patient outcomes. It should come as no surprise that for many procedures there are relationships between a surgeon's training and patient outcomes as well as a surgeon's volume (how often a surgeon performs an operation) and patient outcomes.

The step-wise approach at the first visit to a doctor will typically be the following:

1. history-taking,
2. physical examination,
3. discussion of the diagnosis or possible diagnoses,
4. discussion of investigations that may be needed, either to confirm the diagnosis or to exclude others, and
5. a discussion of treatment options.

The Colorectal Surgeon follows these steps. Nothing special.

Nothing special in the order of the steps, but for patients with anorectal complaints, the way these steps are handled is *very special.* Both history-taking and especially physical examination require sensitivity and the awareness that patients may be embarrassed to talk about their problem. They may be anxious at the prospect of an anal examination and fearful that it will be painful.

Issues of embarrassment, fearfulness, and anxiety are touched on throughout this book, but for now I want to walk you through the physical examination of the anorectum.

The Physical Examination

Like many Colorectal Surgeons, I examine patients on a table called a "procto table." This is also called the "knee-chest position" (see Figure 2). Just before patients are positioned on the table, they slip their pants (or skirts) and underclothes toward their knees, while the area is draped with a large sheet that has a hole in the centre. The table is raised and tipped slightly forward. There is a nurse in the room throughout the examination.

I tell patients what is about to happen at each step along the way. "No sneak attacks." And I reassure them that if there is pain during the course of the examination, the examination will cease.

The first step of the examination consists of a visual inspection of the anus at rest, at squeezing (the act of holding in a bowel movement), and at straining (the act of pushing out a bowel movement).

If painful anal pathology is not evident from the visual examination, then a digital (i.e., finger) rectal examination can safely begin. The patient is asked to bear down slightly; this relaxes the muscles.

Then the lubricated, gloved index finger is gently advanced into the anus and rectum. Resting and squeezing states are noted. The examining finger then sweeps around the entire circumference of the anus and lower rectum to identify any tender areas or palpable abnormalities. The prostate gland, sitting in front of the rectum in men, is checked for irregularities.

Figure 2
A Procto Table

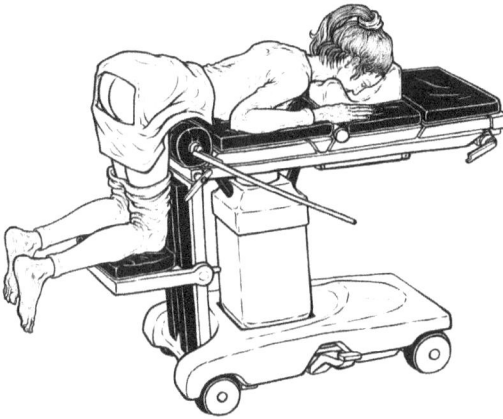

Following visual and digital examination, the anorectum is examined endoscopically – that is, a small scope, commonly called a "proctoscope," is placed into the anus. The scope can usually be advanced as far as the top of the rectum (about 16 cm). The scope has a light source and an insufflation bulb that is used to blow some air into the rectum, separating the rectal walls and allowing direct inspection. Unfortunately, the scope and air produce the sensation of needing to move the bowels, *but that is not happening,* and the feeling disappears when the scope is removed.

And that's it. As the table is lowered the lubricating jelly is wiped away and the patient gets off of the table. I can say that

The anorectal examination is somewhat unpleasant and completely tolerable.

100% of patients find the anorectal examination somewhat unpleasant and completely tolerable. It takes less than 5 minutes. In fact, patients regularly remark on how quick and easy it was.

The Discussion

After the history-taking and examination, I discuss the diagnosis or presumptive diagnosis. I review the problem and its natural history. We may talk about the need for further investigation. I review the treatment options, the recommended treatment, the rationale for the recommendation, the expectations, and potential complications.

I draw pictures explaining the relevant anatomy, their problem, and the treatment options. Nowadays, patients will often take a photo of my artwork. I also give pamphlets to my patients about their diagnosis.

I mainly use the excellent pamphlets that are produced by the ASCRS (American Society of Colon and Rectal Surgeons). The ASCRS has produced pamphlets on almost every conceivable diagnosis and I have all of them in my clinic. I don't let the take-home reading replace *in-class teaching*, but I hope that the pamphlets serve as a reminder of our discussion.

Doctors know that patient retention of the information provided in the clinic is incomplete. I love it when patients are accompanied by a friend or family member – a witness and an accessory memory device. Some patients want to tape our discussion, and that's OK with me.

The Consent Process

If I am recommending an operation or procedure, no matter how small it may seem, I ensure that the four principles of the consent process have been applied. Three of the four principles are addressed with the patient in the clinic: *voluntary, informed,* and *capacity.* I address the fourth principle on my own: *documented.* I make sure to document the meeting and the consent process on the day of the visit to my clinic.

Voluntary means no coercion. *Capacity* means the ability to understand the diagnosis and the management plan, as well as the implications of undergoing or foregoing treatment. Pretty straightforward.

Informed ... the meaning is less clear. I think it means that the patient understands these points.

- The natural history of the disease, that is, what are the likely outcomes if they do nothing about the problem. (I am pretty careful to preface comments about the future with a disclaimer that I don't have a crystal ball, but that predictions are based on evidence and experience.)

- The treatment options, especially the non-operative options.

- The expectations, outcomes, and complications of the treatment options.

- My rationale for making a particular treatment recommendation, including the details of the procedure, the reasonable expectations, and the *potential complications.*

The potential complications? This is where informed gets tricky. Every conceivable complication? Just the common ones? Just the really dangerous and potentially fatal ones? Just the ones that I think that particular patient would want to know?

A guiding principle is *what would a reasonable person want to know in order to decide to undergo or forego a treatment.*

Another guiding principle is *the less essential the treatment, the higher the standard for ensuring that the patient has this knowledge.*

I spend as much time talking to one patient about their hemorrhoids as I spend talking to another about their rectal cancer. The treatment of rectal cancer is almost always mandatory. The treatment of hemorrhoids is almost never mandatory. The reasonable patient with a rectal cancer will invariably accept the recommended treatment and its potential complications. The patient with hemorrhoids may reasonably decline the recommended treatment and the exposure to the potential complications.

Most patients who see me are prepared to make a decision about management right then and there. I don't insist that they go home to think it over. But I do like it when they decide to do so.

1

"I See Blood"

Carol is a 52-year-old woman who came to see me about rectal bleeding. She is on an anti-hypertensive (blood pressure) medication. She has had two uncomplicated vaginal deliveries. Other than high blood pressure, Carol has no medical problems.

Carol describes bright red blood with bowel movements (BM) off and on for about 12 months. For the past 10-12 weeks there has been blood with almost every BM. The blood is mainly on the toilet paper but may also appear on the outside of the stool and may occasionally drip into the bowl.

There has been no dark or clotted blood. She has one formed stool per day; occasionally there is hard stool and straining. There is no pain with defecation. She does have the feeling of tissue protruding at the anus that may be pushed back in when wiping. She is continent for stool and gas (there are no unwanted or unexpected escapes). There has been no change in her bowel habits. There are no complaints of abdominal pain. There is no history of colorectal cancer in her family.

Carol said that she delayed coming to see me because she was embarrassed and afraid, but her symptoms are getting worse and she is worried that she might have colon cancer.

Carol allowed me to proceed with the anorectal examination, including proctoscopy.

She tolerated the examination very well. She was very pleasantly surprised at how quick and painless it was. It was also less embarrassing than she thought it would be.

Carol's history and physical examination revealed grade III mixed hemorrhoids. She asked me, "What does that mean? Why do I have this problem? What can be done about it? Are you sure I don't have cancer?"

WHAT IS A HEMORRHOID?

Hemorrhoid. Great word! Rhoid is sphere. Heme is blood. A hemorrhoid is not exactly a ball of blood. But it's close. A hemorrhoid is a cushion-like thickening of tissue in the upper anal canal filled with blood vessels.

Most people are surprised to learn that these cushions are normal structures. (See Figure 3.) We are born with them – usually three of them. There is a typical distribution of these cushions, one on the left and two on the right, but there is considerable variation.

Most people are surprised to learn that we are born with hemorrhoids – usually three of them.

Because hemorrhoids are normal structures, I make a distinction between hemorrhoids and hemorrhoidal *disease* – that is, hemorrhoids that are causing symptoms.

The hemorrhoidal cushions are suspended by delicate muscle fibres in the upper anal canal. These suspensory fibres can weaken, allowing the cushions to descend and protrude. The blood vessels *within* the cushions stretch and become thin-walled. The displaced cushions, subjected to trauma by the passage of stool, may bleed.

Figure 3

Internal Hemorrhoids

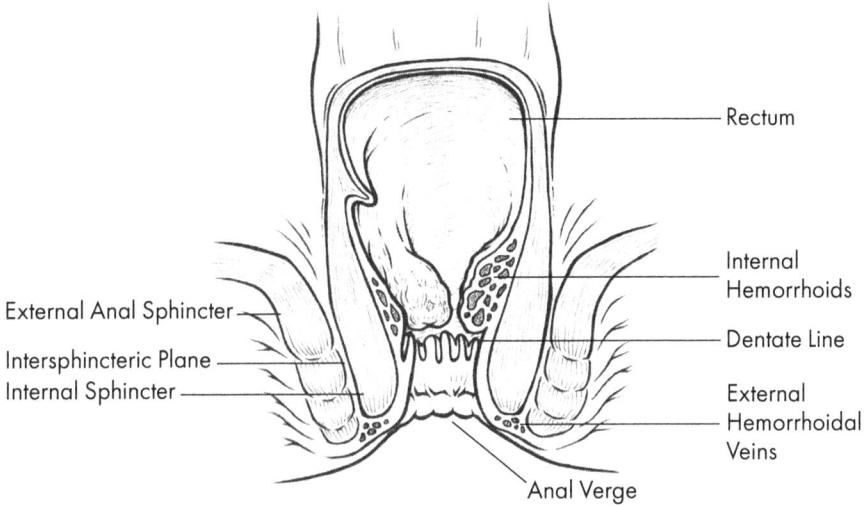

Rectum

Internal Hemorrhoids

Dentate Line

External Hemorrhoidal Veins

External Anal Sphincter

Intersphincteric Plane

Internal Sphincter

Anal Verge

Hemorrhoidal disease, in other words, results from a failure of the suspensory mechanism. It is hypothesized that when our distant ancestors adopted an upright posture, the suspensory fibres could not handle the gravitational strain.

Less far-reaching hypotheses for hemorrhoidal disease are constipation, straining, pregnancy, vaginal delivery, heavy lifting, and squats at the gym. The negative impact of straining and hard stools is easily understood. Just sitting on the toilet for long periods places some strain on the hemorrhoids. Reading on the toilet is a particularly bad idea. I've heard it said that a man's idea of multi-tasking is pooping and reading at the same time. One of my teachers used to offer great advice. He'd tell his patients, "Don't read in the bathroom and don't crap in the library."

But the precise cause of hemorrhoidal disease is still not well understood. For some people, hemorrhoidal disease seems to run in the family. Many hemorrhoid sufferers have no identifiable risk factors – other than their upright posture.

SYMPTOMS AND ASSESSMENT

The most common symptoms of hemorrhoids are bleeding and protrusion.

Bleeding is bright red and painless. Bright red because the blood is oxygenated arterial blood; painless because the hemorrhoidal cushions are inside the body where nerves are *duller*.

A word about *inside/dull* versus *outside/sensitive*. The red-coloured lining of the rectum, called "mucosa," meets the skin of the buttock in about the middle of the anal canal. The junction of mucosa and skin – inside and outside – is marked by an irregular line. Some early anatomist thought the line looked like a row of teeth and named it the "dentate line." Not what I would have gone with frankly, but here we are.

When it comes to anal sensation and pain, the dentate line is very important. Above the dentate line are the kinds of nerves and receptors that run to and from the body's internal organs. These are called "visceral" nerves. Below the dentate line, by contrast, are body wall or "somatic" nerves. The former are, by and large, quite dull, whereas the latter are highly sensitive.

Bleeding appears with bowel movements and, as with Carol, may be seen on the toilet paper, on the outside of the stool, and even dripping, occasionally spraying, into the bowl.

Other diseases of the anus and rectum may be associated with bright red rectal bleeding, notably anal fissure (see Chapter 2) and rectal cancer (see Chapter 8), but dripping into the toilet bowl (or onto the floor!) is highly suggestive of hemorrhoids. Clotted blood, dark blood, and blood mixed with stools suggests a bleeding source in the rectum or left colon and should never be ascribed to hemorrhoids without further investigation.

Protrusion, also called "prolapse," is the other common symptom of hemorrhoidal disease, and may be associated with discomfort, although rarely pain. When protrusion is substantial, the cushions may need to be pushed back in or, in the most advanced pattern of disease, may not go back in. Protrusion may be severe enough that mucous, bloody, and fecal staining of the underclothes may ensue. There may be itch and irritation, but not usually.

Grading Hemorrhoids

Hemorrhoids are graded or staged based on their degree of protrusion and whether they spontaneously reduce *(go back in)*, need to be pushed back in *(manual reduction)* or stay out in a prolapsed position *(irreducible)*. (See Figure 4.) The system helps guide physicians to the appropriate therapeutic option.

Figure 4

Grading of Hemorrhoids

Stage or Grade	Treatment
I (bleeding, no protrusion)	Good bowel habits (this applies to all stages)
II (protrusion, spontaneous reduction)	Rubber Band Ligation
III (protrusion, manual reduction)	Rubber Band Ligation & Hemorrhoid Surgery
IV (protrusion, chronically prolapsed)	Hemorrhoidectomy

For all its benefits, the staging system is only a rough guide to treatment. A major weakness of the system, for instance, is that it ignores size. A grade II hemorrhoid could actually be *larger* than a grade IV hemorrhoid. The grading system also ignores the main determinant of treatment: how much do the hemorrhoids bother the patient?

The grading system also describes *internal* hemorrhoids only.

Mixed Hemorrhoids

Until now, we have been talking solely about internal hemorrhoids, the cushions that are covered by the mucosa (lining of the anus above the dentate line). Carol, however, has mixed hemorrhoids, a combination of internal and external.

This is where things get fussy.

Basically, if it's covered with mucosa rather than skin, it's an internal hemorrhoid, regardless of whether the tissue is inside the anal canal or protruding to the outside world. If the prominent bit of tissue is covered by skin, however, it is an external hemorrhoid, also called a "skin tag."

Tags may be associated with internal hemorrhoidal disease (i.e., mixed hemorrhoids); they may be associated with other anal disease like chronic anal fissure (see Chapter 2); or they may be independent agents.

Unlike internal hemorrhoids, external hemorrhoidal skin tags are not part of normal human anatomy. Tags may be asymptomatic or may cause hygiene or cosmetic issues. But skin tags don't bleed and usually don't cause pain. Itch and irritation may be due to skin tags, but tags are notorious for being innocent bystanders.

On visual inspection of the anus, findings range from normal (i.e., no hemorrhoids) to a cauliflower of hemorrhoidal tissue protruding from the anus – internal, external, or mixed. As I described in an earlier section (When You See a Colorectal Surgeon), the inspection phase of the physical examination includes a request for the patient to strain as if trying to have a BM, which may produce the internal hemorrhoids in patients with grade II or III disease.

Digital rectal findings are generally normal (i.e., the hemorrhoids are not usually felt), although an experienced examiner might appreciate a soft, fleshy fullness.

The scoping phase of the examination provides an excellent look at the hemorrhoids. The degree to which the hemorrhoids bulge into the end of the scope provides a clue regarding the grade of the hemorrhoids.

COLONOSCOPY? REQUIRED FOR HEMORRHOIDS?

When there has been rectal bleeding, doctors have traditionally asked themselves, "Is colonoscopy indicated?" Colonoscopy is the direct visual examination of the entire colon using a 160 cm flexible scope called a "colonoscope."

Behind this question is the recognition that medical history, physical examination, and even proctoscopy (examination with the rigid short scope that only goes a few inches into the rectum) cannot determine with certainty where blood is coming from. Since everyone has hemorrhoidal tissue in the anus, hemorrhoids are highly susceptible to *innocent bystander error*, taking the blame when a more ominous disease upstream of the anus, such as a polyp or cancer, may be the true culprit.

> *The question shouldn't be "Is colonoscopy indicated?" but "Can colonoscopy be deferred?"*

Under these circumstances, the question shouldn't be "Is colonoscopy indicated?" but "Can colonoscopy be deferred?" And I say yes to deferral only if the criteria below are met.

- The patient is under 40 years of age.
- There is no personal history of polyps or cancer of the colon or rectum.
- There is no history of colon or rectal cancer in first-degree relatives (parents, siblings).
- There is no associated inflammatory bowel disease (no history of ulcerative colitis or Crohn's disease).
- There are no unexplained symptoms like change in bowel habits, abdominal pain, weight loss, or fatigue.
- There is no anemia (low hemoglobin).
- A source for blood is found on anorectal examination.
- The blood is exclusively bright red, not dark or clotted, and not mixed with the stool.

▪ The bleeding stops with treatment of the anal pathology.

When all of these conditions are met, I defer colonoscopy. Otherwise, I take a look. I have seen many patients whose lives have probably been saved because I was reluctant to blame the hemorrhoids until the colon had been examined.

Colonoscopy is possible because of flexible fiberoptic technology. The scopes can be guided around corners and can project an image onto a screen. The technology has allowed the development of flexible instruments that can be guided into hollow structures all over the body. Urologists, Gynecologists, Ear, Nose, and Throat Surgeons, Respirologists, and Gastroenterologists all use scopes. Where there is a hole, there is a flexible fiberoptic scope made to go in it. Orthopaedic surgeons actually make holes to put scopes into joints.

The colonoscope can be advanced through the entire colon and right into the small bowel. A channel within the colonoscope allows the operator to pass forceps for taking biopsies and snares that can snip off polyps – a colonoscopic polypectomy (see Figure 5).

Figure 5

Colonoscopic Polypectomy

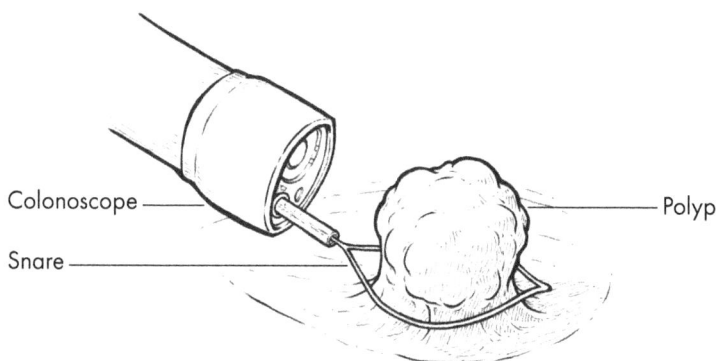

Because it can be uncomfortable, colonoscopy is usually done under sedation. Sedation makes it a very tolerable examination.

The great majority of patients have no pain and often do not even have any discomfort. In fact, the complaints about colonoscopy are almost always directed at *the prep*.

The prep, short for bowel preparation, is the cleaning out of the bowel that must take place in order to get a good look at the colon. Bowel preparation, usually done the day before the procedure, involves a clear fluid diet for about 24 hours as well as drinking a solution that creates watery diarrhea, emptying the colon of its content. It is unpleasant. But most patients find it tolerable.

Colonoscopy is very safe. Even with the removal of polyps, the risk of a severe injury (perforation) is much less than 1 in 500.

HOW ARE HEMORRHOIDS TREATED?

As for the treatment of hemorrhoids, there are two main considerations to determine the best course of action:

1. the stage of the disease, and
2. how much they bother the patient.

Stage doesn't matter if the hemorrhoids aren't impacting the patient's quality of life. But if the patient is fed up and wants treatment, treatment will usually be guided by the stage of the disease.

I offer three treatments for hemorrhoids: conservative management, rubber band ligation, and hemorrhoidectomy (surgical removal). There are other treatments out there, including oral medications that strengthen blood vessels and decrease bleeding, but these three are the treatments with the best supporting evidence and the ones that I have found to be most effective.

Conservative Management

Conservative management is the most common method of treatment. Basically, it means promoting good bowel habits to reduce hard stools and straining.

This remedy includes upping your dietary fibre and fluid intake, maintaining an active lifestyle, cutting out reading on the toilet, and avoiding over-hygienic behaviour – clean is good, but hyper-clean is not good (anal polishing, as it's called, can lead to skin damage, irritation, and itch – see Chapter 3).

Clean is good, but hyper-clean is not good.

For some hemorrhoid sufferers, minimizing or eradicating hard stools and straining can be easily achieved via these established management techniques. For others, especially individuals with irritable bowel syndrome (IBS), grappling with hard stools and straining can be a lifelong and miserable struggle.

Either way, these conservative principles are an essential part of hemorrhoid management, regardless of the stage of disease.

You may have noticed that I have not talked about over-the-counter (OTC) treatments for hemorrhoids. There is a big world of topical lotions, oral potions, suppositories, and wipes. I use them very selectively. The quality of the evidence for these products is poor.

There is no ointment or suppository that can make hemorrhoids go away.

And what symptoms are the ointments targeting? Protrusion? Bleeding? Itch and irritation? Ointments and wipes cannot have a significant or lasting impact on bleeding or protrusion, the main symptoms of hemorrhoidal disease.

Ointments may be soothing, reducing itch and irritation, but these symptoms are more likely due to pruritus ani, not hemorrhoids. And as you will read in Chapter 3 on pruritus ani, ointments, especially those with a steroid or anesthetic agent, can be damaging to the perianal skin.

There is a family of oral agents, called "flavonoids," that have what is called a "phlebotomic" effect, strengthening blood vessels. When bleeding is the main symptom, these medications may help. I have been less impressed with their impact on the other symptoms of hemorrhoidal disease.

Rubber Band Ligation (RBL)

After conservative management, the next-most common treatment is rubber band ligation (RBL). To ligate is to tie up, which means that the proximal end of the hemorrhoid (i.e., the end closest to the rectum) is tied by a tight rubber band. It takes less than 5 minutes and is not painful when done correctly.

To conduct RBL, a small scope is placed in the anal canal, the patient is asked to strain so that the hemorrhoids bulge, and then a special applicator gun suctions some of the hemorrhoidal tissue into the barrel of the gun. The operator confirms that the patient is not having any pain and then the gun is *fired*, pushing two tight elastic bands onto the tissue. Two bands in case one breaks. The bands literally strangle the incorporated tissue, which shrivels and falls off over the next 3-10 days, leaving a wound that heals over the following few weeks. The banding destroys some hemorrhoidal tissue, but more importantly, it produces scar tissue that anchors the cushion in the upper anus where it belongs.

Patients may feel some discomfort for a day or two, but by taking care to test sensation before firing, pain should occur in less than 1% of patients. Needing to remove a band due to pain is very rare.

Complications are also rare. Bleeding, for instance, may occur from the wound between 3 and 10 days after banding, but the rate of this complication is less than 1%. Infection has also been reported and can be very serious, but the rate is less than 1/10,000, maybe less than 1/100,000. Banding is so common and infection so incredibly rare that the exact incidence is unknown. I have never seen a post-banding infection in over 40 years of practice.

Most patients need two to three sites banded to achieve symptom control. Some surgeons will do two or three sites at a time. I prefer to do only one hemorrhoid, the worst one, at the first visit. I arrange follow-up in 4 weeks. At the second visit, assuming the patient tolerated the first banding well, and if symptoms warrant, I will offer banding of more than one site at the second session.

When it comes to the results of banding, the expression "You get what you pay for" seems to apply. Banding is a simple office procedure with essentially no recovery period. Patients leave the clinic immediately after banding and return to normal life with only three instructions.

1. Avoid hard stools and straining for at least 2 weeks.
2. Don't take blood thinners. (Some patients will need to interrupt their blood thinner prescription in order to have banding.)
3. Call me if you are having any difficulties.

For this small investment you get a modest 70% likelihood of significant improvement. Improvement is reasonably durable. Some touch-up banding is done in 20-30% of patients.

Banding works best for grade II and small grade III hemorrhoids. Because of the pain that would be involved, bands unfortunately cannot be applied to external hemorrhoids, so if the external component is thought to be a significant contributor to the patient's symptoms, one of the other treatment options should be considered.

Hemorrhoidectomy

Excision, or cutting out the hemorrhoids, *hemorrhoidectomy,* is the third option. By surgical standards, it is a great operation. The success rate is very high; the complication rate is very low. Over 90% of patients are very pleased with the results of the operation, and complications like bleeding, infection, and diminished continence are all in the 1% range. The wounds can be slow to heal but do heal very nicely.

So why does hemorrhoidectomy have a terrible reputation? In a word, pain. It is a miserable operation in terms of post-operative pain, and all the local anesthetic, pain-killers, laxatives, tub baths, and topicals can't seem to change that. The wounds, often three of them, are in a terribly sensitive part of the body, plus the anal sphincter muscles and pelvic floor muscles respond with spasm, adding to the pain. And the combination of constipating analgesics (pain-killers) and spastic muscles, make it hard to have a soft bowel movement without straining.

In addition to difficulty passing stool after hemorrhoidectomy, a more immediate problem is difficulty passing urine. Urinary retention is the result of spasm of the pelvic floor muscles, including the urinary sphincter. Pain-killers and anesthetic agents can also contribute to this complication. Warm tub baths and peeing in the tub may solve the problem. Some patients will need an *in and out catheterization* of the bladder before discharge home from the recovery area. (*In and out* means a catheter is passed *in* to empty the bladder, but once emptied, the catheter is taken *out* of the bladder.) We try to reduce the frequency of this problem by having the patient pee before the operation and restricting intra-venous fluid administration during the operation.

There's no doubt about it, it's a tough road to recovery. At least 2 weeks before patients feel human again, and closer to 2-3 months before patients can fully put the operation behind them. Pun intended.

That is why a painless, effective treatment for hemorrhoidal disease is the Holy Grail of colorectal surgery. Unfortunately, to be painless, the treatment has to be applied above the dentate line, and by being applied above the dentate line, efficacy is compromised.

As I mentioned, patient satisfaction with hemorrhoidectomy is well over 90%, but I make sure that patients understand that satisfaction and perfection are not the same and that the latter is much less likely. The reason that the results tend to be less than perfect is two-fold.

First, we do not remove *all* of the hemorrhoidal tissue. We remove the main hemorrhoids, but if we are overly aggressive, trying to remove every bit of the hemorrhoidal cushions, then we risk taking away too much tissue. Excessive removal results in something called "anal stenosis" – a tight anus, an opening that is too small. Anal stenosis can be solved, but it is much better to avoid it in the first place. A droll wisecrack among Colorectal Surgeons is, "When patients with anal stenosis pass gas, only dogs can hear it."

Second, the skin around the anus, *the perianal skin,* may swell, and healing may be associated with minor degrees of tag formation. The tags or external hemorrhoids are usually small and not bothersome, but I warn patients about this potential complication.

IT'S JUST HEMORRHOIDS? NOT CANCER?

Carol asked me if I was sure she didn't have colon cancer. This is a common question.

I reassured Carol that it was very unlikely she had colon cancer. Her symptoms, including exclusively bright red blood, as well as the physical findings, pointed very convincingly to hemorrhoidal disease.

Nevertheless, I recommended she have a colonoscopy to rule out the possibility of colorectal cancer, and I did so for three main reasons.

1. Colorectal cancer is common. There is about a 4% risk of developing this disease by the age of 75, making it one of the most common cancers. The rate starts going up around age 40 and keeps on rising. And Carol, recall, is 52.
2. Colon cancer has cure rates in the range of 90% when found in its early stages.
3. Colon cancer has a precursor lesion called a polyp. Removing polyps during colonoscopy prevents colon cancer. Polyps are very common; about 20-30% of us over age 50 have polyps. Once identified as a polyp grower, patients should have colonoscopy at regular intervals. The frequency of examinations is guided by how many polyps are identified, but a typical interval is every 5 years.

Carol was fed up with her symptoms. She elected to proceed with colonoscopy and hemorrhoidectomy.

The colonoscopy revealed that in addition to mixed hemorrhoids, Carol had sigmoid diverticulosis and two small polyps, 5 mm and 8 mm in size, one in the ascending colon and one in the rectum. The polyps were removed with a snare and sent to the pathology department. These were both tubular adenomas (benign growths).

POLYPS

Carol and I talked about the polyps and the diverticulosis.

Polyp is not a very specific term. It refers to a protrusion into the lumen, the central cavity of a hollow organ like the colon. There are several types of polyps, but the important ones are abnormal growths that arise from the lining (the mucosa) of the bowel.

The growths, called "adenomas" or "adenomatous polyps," are benign. They do not have the potential to invade into other tissues or to spread (metastasize) to other organs. But as adenomas get bigger, some will become malignant. They are now called "carcinomas." This progression is called the "polyp-cancer" or "adenoma-carcinoma" sequence. The sequence is interrupted by removing polyps.

Colonoscopy is extremely good at finding and safely removing polyps. Once a patient is identified as a grower of adenomas, it is recommended that they have surveillance colonoscopies. A common surveillance program is to have colonoscopy at 5-year intervals.

Once identified as a polyp grower, surveillance colonoscopies are recommended.

Carol and I talked about the polyps and when the pathology report came back, I let her know that these were benign polyps called adenomas and that no additional treatment was needed. I reviewed with her that there was a risk that she might grow more polyps and that a surveillance program of colonoscopy every 5 years was a good idea. Carol was concerned that 5 years was too long between examinations, but I assured her that it was actually an extremely safe regimen to follow.

DIVERTICULOSIS

Diverticula are pockets or out-pouchings that project from the walls of hollow organs like the colon. (They do not appear in solid organs like the liver or the kidneys.) The most common kind of diverticula in the gastrointestinal (GI) tract are those arising in the sigmoid colon (see Figure 6).

In Western countries, more than half of us over the age of 50 develop sigmoid diverticula. It is thought that this is because of our diets being low in fibre. Low dietary fibre results in hard stools and high intra-colonic pressure that is thought to push the colonic lining (mucosa) out through the colonic muscle wall. This hypothesis is likely to be at least part of the story, but the cause of diverticula is not fully understood.

The presence of diverticula in the colon is called "diverticulosis." Diverticulosis causes no symptoms unless a diverticulum bleeds or becomes infected. Bleeding is rare but infection, called "diverticulitis," is relatively common. Diverticulitis is caused by the bacteria that live in the colon. The risk of developing diverticulitis is in the range of 5-10%. Diverticulitis causes abdominal pain and may be associated with bloating, change in bowel habits, and features of infection like fever, chills, and sweats.

The human GI tract contains many trillions of bacteria. This enormous family of bugs, primarily in the colon, is called the "gut microbiome." The microbiome plays a critical role in human health ... and disease. The bacteria of the microbiome perform essential activities in digestion, nutrition, and immunology. But they are also responsible for appendicitis, diverticulitis, and anal abscess-fistula (Chapter 4) and are implicated in many other diseases, including irritable bowel syndrome, inflammatory bowel disease (Chapter 11), obesity, and even heart disease, to name a few. Manipulation of the gut microbiome to improve human health is the subject of intense scientific investigation.

Diverticulitis almost always settles without the need for emergency operation, but some people will experience recurrent attacks, leading to a recommendation for scheduled, sometimes called "elective," surgery to resect (remove) the involved segment of the colon. The bowel ends are then reconnected; the connection is called an "anastomosis."

Complications from diverticulitis may also lead to a recommendation for sigmoid resection. The two most common complications are *fistula* and *stricture.*

A fistula is an abnormal connecting tunnel with another organ. The most common organ to be the *passive recipient* or *innocent-bystander* of fistula from sigmoid diverticulitis is the bladder. The floppy sigmoid segment of colon can lie right next to the bladder within the pelvis. The inflammation of diverticulitis can damage the thin bladder wall and create a communication between the sigmoid colon and the bladder, a *colovesical fistula.* Colonic bacteria enter the bladder resulting in recurrent urinary tract infections. Gas and stool can even enter resulting in fecaluria (bits of stool in the urine) and pneumaturia (bubbles of colonic gas in the urine). Fistula will invariably lead to a decision for operation.

Figure 6

Sigmoid Diverticulosis

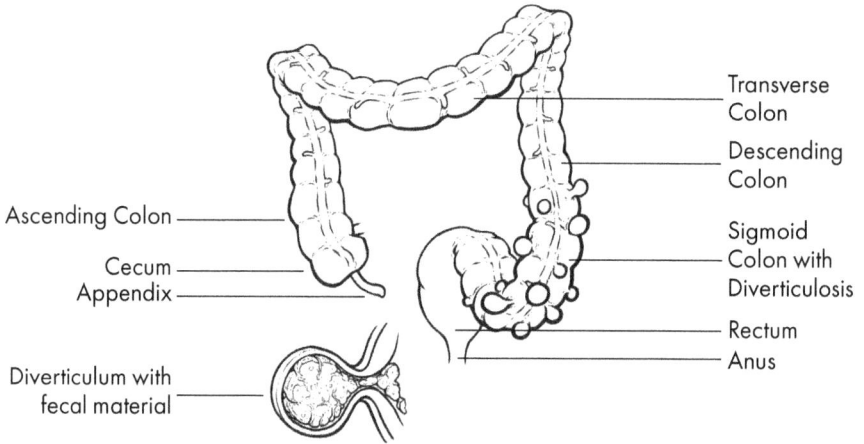

Transverse Colon

Descending Colon

Sigmoid Colon with Diverticulosis

Rectum

Anus

Ascending Colon

Cecum

Appendix

Diverticulum with fecal material

Women who have had a hysterectomy can develop a *colo-vaginal fistula* in the same way. The thick-walled uterus is virtually never affected by fistula, but if the uterus is not there to *protect* the vagina, sigmoid diverticulitis can create a communication with the vagina leading to horrible symptoms and the need for operation.

A stricture is a narrowing of the colonic lumen (channel). A stricture may develop when inflammation creates scar tissue in the colonic wall. Colonic strictures cause obstructive symptoms like cramping, bloating, and irregular bowel function. This complication may also lead to scheduled resection.

The most common cause of obstruction of the colon, however, isn't diverticulitis or other forms of inflammation. It is cancer of the colon. When a patient has episodes of new abdominal pain, bloating, and a change in bowel habits, colon cancer is the disease that must be ruled out. Colonoscopy will lead to the diagnosis.

Carol and I talked about the diverticula (diverticulosis) and that her risk of developing infection of the diverticula, called diverticulitis, was less than 10%. The symptoms of diverticulitis and its natural history were reviewed, as were the possible protective effects of a high-fibre diet. *Contrary to popular belief, there was no need for Carol to avoid seeds and nuts.*

Carol had a three-quadrant hemorrhoidectomy a few weeks after the colonoscopy. The pre-op orders for Carol were nothing to eat or drink for 6 hours prior to the scheduled start of the operation, and one Fleet enema 2-3 hours before leaving for the hospital. The three main cushions and their associated tags were excised. The operation was done under general anesthesia (GA). Carol was offered epidural anesthesia but she preferred the GA approach.

The sphincter muscles were identified during the operative removal of the hemorrhoidal cushions and were not injured during the dissection.

The operation took 30 minutes. Carol went home about 4 hours later. She started tub baths, laxatives, and analgesics shortly after arriving home.

At follow-up 3 weeks later, Carol was still uncomfortable but much improved. The wounds were healing nicely. A few days earlier, she had returned to work on a part-time basis. She agreed that my warnings about a miserable recovery were correct but that she was already very pleased and that she made the right decision to proceed with the operation. Carol said she'd call in 5 years for follow-up colonoscopy.

At her final follow-up appointment, Carol told me that she wished she hadn't delayed coming to see me. She hadn't come earlier partly because she was embarrassed, but ultimately the severity of her symptoms and a nagging worry that she might have cancer pushed her to overcome her embarrassment. She said that now she feels silly; it wasn't that bad, she is no longer worried about colon cancer, and her hemorrhoids are gone.

"My Bum Hurts"

FISSURE, THROMBOSED EXTERNAL
HEMORRHOID, ABSCESS

Lee is an 18-year-old, first-year university student who came to see me about painful bowel movements he has been experiencing over the past 6 months. Lee is not on any medications and has no significant medical history.

Lee says that when he first moved into his dorm 6 months ago, he had a few weeks of constipation. He describes hard stools every 2-3 days associated with straining, anal pain, and blood. Bowel habits have returned to his usual pattern of one formed stool per day, but pain and blood have persisted. The pain feels like tearing or cutting and may last for minutes to an hour after defecation.

The blood is bright red and appears mainly on the toilet paper and occasionally as a streak on the outside of the stool. He does not push anything "back in" but it feels like "there is a hemorrhoid." He is continent for stool and gas. His family history is negative for bowel diseases.

On examination, there is some pain even with gentle separation of the buttocks. A fissure (a tear in the tissue) can be seen in the posterior midline anoderm (the skin of the lower anal canal, below the dentate line, where the skin meets the mucosa). There is an associated skin tag in the posterior midline. There are no signs of local infection. Because separation of the buttocks was painful, examination was limited to inspection.

Anal pain is a favourite symptom among Colorectal Surgeons. This is because making the correct diagnosis is easy – there are only three common causes of anal pain.

1. Fissure
2. Thrombosed external hemorrhoid
3. Abscess

Each has its own characteristic complaints and physical findings and there are effective treatments for all three.

Let's dive in.

FISSURE

A fissure is a tear in the anoderm, located in either the posterior or anterior midline. The occasional patient who has fissures in *both* anterior and posterior positions is said to have "kissing fissures."

The tear may be caused by hard stools, although not all patients describe this. All patients describe painful defecation, often with a trace of bright blood on the toilet paper and sometimes on the outside of the stool. The pain may fade after a few minutes, but some patients will have pain that lasts for hours. And the pain can be severe.

When a fissure first develops, it looks like a paper cut. This is called an "acute fissure." Over time, fissures become broader, deeper, and develop scar tissue at their edges. As they widen, they become less like a paper cut and more like a pear-shaped or elliptical ulcer. The tissue at either end of the fissure may swell, producing a skin tag (external hemorrhoid) and a hypertrophied anal papilla. This is called a "chronic fissure."

The reason some fissures become chronic, and probably the reason patients get a fissure in the first place, is that fissure patients have anal sphincter spasm. Specifically, the internal anal sphincter is overactive. This is called "hypertonicity."

Hypertonicity is a sustained contraction of the muscle. It is tempting to think that hypertonicity is secondary to the pain of the fissure, but it appears more likely that internal anal sphincter hypertonicity is a pre-existing state in fissure patients. We don't know why.

The increased contraction of the internal anal sphincter muscle results in decreased blood flow to the tissue. Less blood flow means less oxygen delivery. And less oxygen delivery means less healing. The fissure becomes chronic.

How Are Fissures Treated?

The initial treatment for both acute and chronic fissure is directed at the two factors that caused the fissure: trauma (usually hard stools) and spasm.

Moderate physical activity speeds transit through the colon and is associated with good bowel habits.

Acute Fissures

For some patients, good bowel habits may be achieved through a combination of high fibre diet, fibre supplements like psyllium, prunes or prune juice, lots of water, and an active lifestyle. Moderate physical activity speeds transit through the colon and is associated with good bowel habits.

Some patients need to use laxatives.

For the record, I do not recommend laxatives like senna and herbal teas. These *stimulant* laxatives work by causing contraction of the muscles in the wall of the colon. They are very effective, but with prolonged use the colonic muscles stop responding to the stimulation. The result is a lazy bowel ... and worsening constipation.

Stimulant laxatives, especially products containing senna or cascara, produce *melanosis coli,* a brown or black pigmentation of the colonic lining that can be seen during colonoscopy. It is a completely harmless condition and has no relationship to the development of polyps or cancer. The pigmentation slowly fades away after cessation of the laxative.

Instead, I favour the polyethylene glycol (PEG) products. PEG laxatives allow patients to adjust the dose to their individual needs. PEG is usually well tolerated and, unlike the stimulant laxatives, it does not produce a lazy bowel that requires ever-increasing doses.

Internal anal sphincter hypertonicity is attacked in two ways.

Warm tub baths, or sitz baths, cause relaxation of the internal anal sphincter (reduced tone), improving blood flow, and encouraging fissure healing. The effect of a tub bath on the sphincter appears to last for the duration of the bath and for about 30 minutes afterwards. Two or three baths per day are recommended. They are particularly soothing after a bowel movement (BM).

The second way of relaxing the sphincter is by applying medications directly to the anus. Nitric oxide, for instance, is a neurotransmitter that inhibits sphincter muscle contraction. Delivering nitric oxide to the sphincter by applying nitroglycerine ointment (NTG) on the perianal skin (skin around the anus) will result in the healing of some fissures.

NTG, however, causes headaches in many patients, and has largely been replaced by ointments containing a calcium-channel blocker, either diltiazem or nifedipine. These medications also inhibit contraction.

Fortunately, the drop in anal pressure caused by these topical agents is insufficient to affect continence. In other words, patients do not start experiencing unwanted escape of gas or stool when using one of these products.

More than 80% of acute fissures heal with the conservative management described above. Unfortunately, once fissures become chronic, these measures work for fewer than half of patients. The best next step is controversial.

Chronic Fissures

The competing treatment options for chronic fissures are the following:

1. the injection of Botox™ into the sphincter,
2. closure of the fissure with a skin flap, and
3. an operation called "lateral internal sphincterotomy" (LIS).

LIS has by far the highest rate of fissure healing, but LIS results in a permanent decrease in resting pressure (internal anal sphincter contraction) and this is associated with a small risk of minor incontinence. I tend to use the Botox™ or flap approaches when the risk of incontinence appears to be increased, for example, in patients who have a tendency to frequent, loose stools, who have imperfect continence for flatus (gas), or who have had difficult vaginal deliveries.

When Botox™ is used, it is injected right into the sphincter muscle to lower tone (decrease contraction of the sphincter), increase blood flow, and encourage fissure healing. Patients may experience a minor degree of incontinence for gas, but the effect wears off within 2 to 3 months. My personal experience with this approach has been disappointing, with only about 50% of patients achieving durable fissure healing. Botox™ can be repeated and it burns no bridges. Other than very minor and transient incontinence for gas, it is complication-free.

Closure with a skin flap is my least favourite treatment for fissure. In this operation, a flap of skin and subcutaneous fat is dissected at the anal margin (the zone around the opening to the anus) and the flap is sutured (stitched) over the fissure as a patch. The flap brings its own blood supply with it. Success is in the range of 70-80%, but it is a much more painful operation than LIS, has a longer recovery time, and the *donor* site can be slow to heal. But the flap operation has no impact on continence and it is popular among some surgeons.

I think LIS, lateral internal sphincterotomy, represents the best balance of risks and benefits for the patients who do not respond to conservative management. The operation is the division of a short length of the internal anal sphincter muscle. The muscle division reliably produces a drop in sphincter tone, an increase in blood flow (oxygen delivery), and fissure healing in about 95% of patients.

I prefer to do LIS in the operating room under a brief general anesthetic (the patient is asleep) or regional anesthetic (the patient is frozen below the waist). I do what is called a "closed" LIS in which a tiny blade, closer to a needle than a scalpel, is inserted into the groove between the internal anal sphincter (IAS) and external anal sphincter (EAS). The blade then cuts the IAS. The skin wound is so tiny that it doesn't need to be closed with a stitch. The length of muscle division is roughly 1 cm. I tailor the length of the division to the length of the sphincter. A big man gets a longer LIS than a tiny woman.

It is a very well tolerated operation. Patients go home a few hours after the operation and return to regular life within a day or two. Although the fissure may take a couple of weeks to fully heal, hypertonicity is immediately interrupted and fissure pain resolves almost as quickly. The complications of infection and bleeding are about 1% each. As for the risk of incontinence, the story is a bit more complicated.

Humans are tremendously fond of continence, both on the urinary and fecal sides. Loss of continence is distressing. It can be life-ruining. As a general rule, operations that put continence at risk are best avoided.

So, when it comes to LIS, how big is the risk and how bad is the incontinence?

We are not talking about diapers, pads, staining of the underclothes, or surprises. (One of my teachers liked to refer to such surprises as "a fart with a lump in it.") In my opinion, we are not even talking about a degree of urgency with the need to have a BM. My experience with LIS is that, *when specifically asked about it,* 5-10% of patients may describe less perfect control of flatus.

I have to disclose that my personal observations on the safety of LIS may under-estimate the degree or prevalence of incontinence. One reason may be that my patients are so happy to be free of their fissure pain that they don't want to complain. Another reason may be that I avoid LIS in patients whom I suspect to be at increased risk, most notably patients who describe any degree of urgency, incontinence, or tendency to diarrhea, and women who describe long labour and traumatic vaginal delivery. Finally, I do not have a standard length of sphincter division and tailor the operation to the length of the sphincter.

But I have no doubt that for the vast majority of fissure sufferers, the risk-to-benefit ratio with LIS is extremely acceptable and it remains an excellent operation.

By the way, *lateral* means that the division is done *on the side.* Why? The simple answer is that it avoids a wound in the midline. Fissures are in the midline and our surgical forebears learned that making a wound within the fissure is a bad idea. Healing is slower in the midline and a notch may persist at the site, called a "keyhole deformity." The keyhole can be a source of seepage and hygiene problems.

Lee increased the fibre and fluid in his diet and, when he remembered, took a psyllium supplement to soften his stool. He used warm tub baths when he could and he applied a calcium-channel blocker ointment twice daily. He followed up with me in 6 weeks. The symptoms and physical findings were unchanged.

After a review of options and potential complications, Lee elected to proceed with LIS and tag excision.

The operation was done under regional anesthesia (spinal). The chronic anal fissure was identified in the posterior midline of the anal canal. The fissure was examined to assess whether there was a superficial fistula (tunnel) associated with it. Lee did not have a fistula complicating his fissure (about 5% of fissures develop local infection and form a subcutaneous fistula), but he did have a skin tag and a hypertrophied anal papilla. These were excised.

Then the LIS was done, dividing 1 cm of the internal sphincter in the left lateral position. The tiny skin wound was left alone.

At follow-up 3 weeks later, Lee was delighted. He became pain-free a few days after the operation. He had no complaints. When specifically questioned about any decrease in his ability to hold gas, he indicated that there was no change. The fissure was almost fully healed and the LIS wound was barely visible.

LIS is one of my favourite operations. High success, low-risk, happy customers.

THROMBOSED EXTERNAL HEMORRHOID

Anal pain can also be caused by a thrombosed external hemorrhoid (TEH). TEH is a painful and tender lump that forms at the anal verge (at the border between the anus and the buttocks). The name is a bit of a misnomer. It suggests that a "thrombus" or blood clot has formed in a vein at the anal verge, when it is more likely that one of these veins developed a tear, resulting in bleeding into the tissue, creating a tender lump.

TEH results from physical exertion such as heavy lifting or straining at stool. Occasionally, it can develop in the absence of any unusual activity. TEH tends to deliver a steady, severe pain that sends patients to the emergency room (ER) or to their Family

Physician within a day or two. Physical examination reveals a tense, tender, purple lump at the anus.

As for treatment, it is guided by the severity of the symptoms and by the *natural history* of TEH. Natural history is medicalese for what happens to a disease when it is left alone.

The natural history of TEH is favourable. It will resolve on its own. The blood in the tissues breaks up or breaks through the skin. In either case, the release of pressure is accompanied by resolution of pain.

TEH will resolve on its own. Unfortunately, resolution does not happen for at least 4-5 days.

Unfortunately, this resolution does not happen for at least 4-5 days. So, for patients who present within the first few days and who are in significant distress, the approach is excision of the lump. Easily done under local anesthesia in the clinic or ER, the relief is profound and immediate. Most surgeons will leave the small wound open. The wound is minimally painful and heals nicely over the next week or two.

Excision of the TEH not only quickly solves the problem – it prevents the formation of a skin tag that inevitably forms at the site of the TEH.

Since the natural history is one of resolution, patients who are not in significant distress, or who arrive in the clinic after symptoms have started to wane, will be managed conservatively with a mild pain-killer, tub baths, and dietary advice on how to achieve a daily, soft BM.

TEH is not usually a recurrent problem.

ABSCESS

The third possible culprit causing anal pain is abscess. With respect to the suddenness (or acuity) of onset, anal abscess lies somewhere between fissure and thrombosed external hemorrhoid, but is ultimately more like TEH. A patient with an abscess will typically experience several days of worsening, steady pain near the anus. Like TEH, there is no bleeding, but unlike TEH, there is not a discrete lump. Instead, the patient is likely to describe a tender fullness or swelling at or adjacent to the anus. And while the onset of abscess is relatively fast, there is no precipitating event like constipation or heavy lifting. Unlike fissure, the pain of abscess is not closely linked to BMs.

An abscess is a collection of pus – in this case, a collection of pus in one of the *spaces* around the anus. These spaces, located around the anus and rectum, are filled with fatty tissue, blood vessels, lymphatic vessels, and nerves that travel to and from the anorectum and pelvic floor muscles. (See Figure 7.)

Humans have about a dozen glands in the anus, located at the level of the dentate line. As far as I know, none of us are able to use our anal glands to mark our territory or identify one another, like some of our mammalian relatives are able to do.

Figure 7

The Anal Glands and Spaces

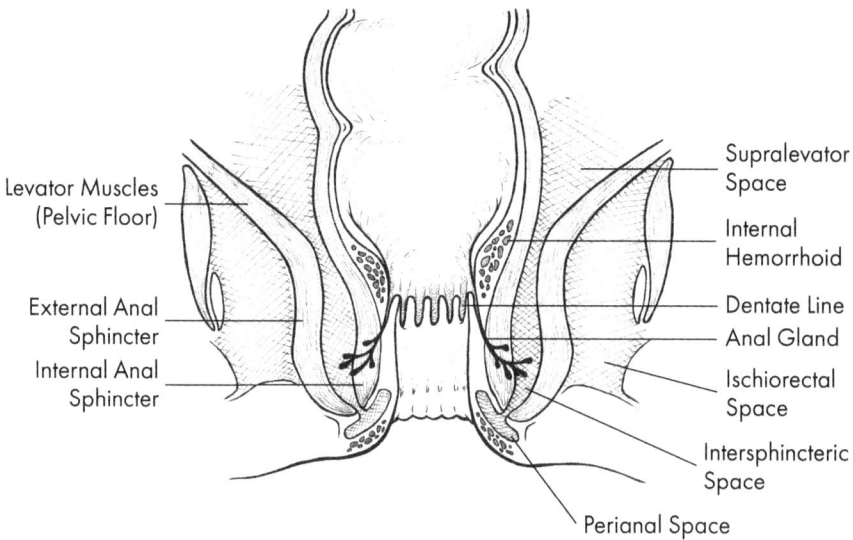

Some of these glands extend into the tissues as far as the space between the sphincters, possibly even to the space beyond the sphincters. These glands can get infected, and when that happens, infected fluid (pus) forms, producing an abscess. The abscess causes pain, fullness, and tenderness. Occasionally, patients may even feel unwell and feverish. Within days of onset, the symptoms are sufficient to prompt a trip to the doctor, often the ER.

Natural history? For the patient who toughs it out, the abscess may ripen and burst through the overlying skin. This spontaneous drainage might not happen for days or weeks. While making its way to the skin, the pus may extend to other spaces, even around to the other side of the anus. When infection tracks to the other side of the anus it is called a "horseshoe" abscess.

In women with infection of an anterior anal gland, the infection can spontaneously drain into the vagina. As we will see in Chapter 6, drainage into the vagina can create a difficult problem.

Because of increasing pain, most patients will not wait for spontaneous drainage to occur. They will seek help and undergo operative drainage. As with the TEH (see earlier in this chapter), this is usually easily accomplished in the clinic or ER under local anesthesia. After freezing the skin, some skin is removed from over the abscess and the pus is drained. The relief is immediate and almost complete.

But before proceeding with drainage of the abscess, there should be a discussion with the patient about the nature of the pathology, its natural history, the treatment options, the recommended treatment, the rationale for the recommendation, and the expectations and potential complications. The discussion of natural history is particularly relevant to anal abscess, because for half of the patients with anal gland infection, draining the abscess is only phase one of their management.

Before draining the abscess, there should be a discussion about the risk of forming a fistula.

After drainage of the abscess 50% of patients will develop a fistula – an abnormal tunnel-like connection between the gland-of-origin and the external drainage site on the skin around the anus. If fistula formation is not discussed with the patient prior to the drainage procedure, the patient who develops a fistula may come to believe that the drainage procedure was not done properly, when, in fact, fistula formation is part of the natural history of abscess, both with and without surgical intervention. Countless times, I have had to divest patients of their conviction that they have a fistula because their surgeon had botched the drainage operation.

If a fistula forms, the patient is likely to experience either on-going drainage or recurrent abscesses. Operative treatment is required to solve the problem. (Fistula management is discussed in Chapter 4.)

What about antibiotics? Traditionally, antibiotics have not been added to incision and drainage (I&D) unless there was a lot of surrounding infection of the skin, called "cellulitis," or if the patient's immunity was thought to be compromised. Recently, there has been some evidence that the addition of antibiotics may decrease the risk of fistula formation, so I now prescribe a 1-week course of antibiotic therapy.

ANAL PAIN POSTSCRIPT

Really? Abscess, fissure, and thrombosed external hemorrhoid. No other causes of anal pain?

OK, I have simplified the pain issue a bit. While these three lesions do account for *almost all* the patients with anal pain, there is the occasional patient with anal pain who does not fit into one of these diagnostic boxes. Two other diseases need to be considered.

Anal cancer can cause pain. Blood with BMs, mucous discharge, itch, discomfort, and "I feel something down there" are earlier and more prominent symptoms of anal cancer, but cancer can also cause pain. If anal tenderness precludes a thorough examination in the clinic, then patients with unexplained anal pain will need to undergo further work-up, usually a combination of MRI (magnetic resonance imaging) and EUA (examination under anaesthesia). If a suspicious lesion is identified at EUA, then it is biopsied (i.e., a piece of tissue is snipped off from the lesion and sent to the pathology department). About 80% of anal cancers are cured by combined chemotherapy and radiotherapy. Anal cancer is discussed in Chapter 8.

Levator syndrome (LS) is a tricky diagnosis. It belongs to an awkward diagnostic category that doctors call *a diagnosis of exclusion* (DOE). DOEs are diagnoses that are left behind after all other diagnoses have been excluded. The key feature of a DOE is that it does not have a test that proves it is correct. The diagnosis is made solely on the basis of symptoms (complaints) and signs (findings on physical examination).

Patients with a DOE often need re-evaluations. Afterall, when a doctor makes a DOE because they have excluded all the other diagnoses, what they have really done is excluded all the other diagnoses *that they could think of.* Not the same thing.

Levator syndrome is a disease with a big clinical spectrum. That's why it's a tricky diagnosis. Men and women. Young and old. It is characterized by anal and/or pelvic pain. The pain may be described as sharp or dull. Severity of the pain can vary. It may be spontaneous or may have triggers. There may or may not be a history of local trauma. It may have relieving factors, or not. Pain may be intermittent or almost continuous. It may last for minutes, hours, or all day. It may awaken patients from sleep. It may or may not have a relationship to BMs, posture, physical activity, stress, or anxiety. It may radiate into the buttocks and thighs or stay in the pelvis. Frequency is also all over the map – daily event or once a year. It can be a minor nuisance or a major disability.

Physical examination may be entirely normal, or there may be tenderness on digital rectal examination when pressure is placed on one or both sides of the pelvic floor muscles (the levators). Sometimes the muscles feel tight on digital rectal exam.

We think that LS is due to spasm (contraction) of the pelvic floor and/or anal sphincter muscles, but why this is happening is uncertain. There is no test that proves that LS is the right diagnosis. A classic DOE.

Many treatments have been tried. I have had most success with a combination of reassurance, pelvic floor physiotherapy, and Botox™ injection of the levators. Unfortunately, the duration of benefit following Botox™ is variable, and I have several patients who return to the clinic at intervals as short as 4-6 months for top-ups. It's worth it to them.

Reassurance as step-one of the therapeutic program may seem a bit patronizing, but it isn't. LS is under-recognized and under-diagnosed. Patients have often been unsuccessfully seeking help from the medical profession for years. Some have been told "there's nothing wrong with you" or "it's all in your head." These patients are pleased to learn that they have *a real disease,* that they are not imagining the symptoms, and that they are not alone. One of my patients with LS suffered so much and for so long that when he comes to my clinic twice per year for a Botox™ shot, he tells my students, "I have hung a picture of Dr. Burnstein in my home right next to my picture of Jesus." (Don't worry, I am completely certain he is joking.)

Proctalgia fugax (PF) is a specific pattern of LS that lasts minutes. The severity of the pain can awaken the patient, typically a young adult, in the middle of the night. Because of PF's characteristic pattern, and the essentially normal physical exanimation, I can make this DOE with more confidence than usual.

Diagnostic Labels

The names we have given to diseases are often not very helpful. Diagnostic labels that have simply converted the patient's chief complaint into Greek or Latin are even a little humiliating. We are fooling no one. Pruritus ani (discussed in Chapter 3) is a classic. The patient complains

of an *itchy bum*, and we diagnose them with *itchy bum* ...
in Latin! Proctalgia fugax (PF) is my personal favourite
from this genre. It is Latin for *fleeting rectal pain*.

A final word about anal pain. Pruritus ani, as we will see in the
next chapter, is a difficult condition characterized by itch and irritation. In its most aggressive forms, PA can be associated with skin
damage that is so severe that patients complain not only of itch,
but of painful erosions, ulceration, and fissures (of the skin, not the
anus). This is not common and the dominant symptoms arising from
the damaged perianal skin are itch and irritation, not pain.

"This Itch Is Driving Me Crazy"

PRURITUS ANI

Michael is a 41-year-old who complains of having "hemorrhoids for about five years." He is bothered by itch and sometimes a burning sensation. It is particularly bad in bed at night. He tries not to scratch but often can't help it. When the itch is at its worst, he may see a trace of bright red blood on the toilet paper. He is meticulous with hygiene, especially after BMs, when he will use a soapy face cloth to wash the area. He has tried many ointments, including prescriptions from doctors. He is currently using an ointment with a combination of lidocaine and hydrocortisone.

Michael's GI enquiry ("enquiry" is medicalese for a check-list of how a body system is working) reveals one semi-formed stool per day, no hard stool, and minimal straining at evacuation. Bright blood rarely appears on the toilet paper. There is no pain or protrusion with defecation. He describes continence for gas. There is no staining of underclothes.

Michael has no other areas affected by itch. He has no allergies or skin conditions. He is generally healthy but overweight (Body Mass Index 35).

Michael does not take any medications but uses Metamucil® daily.

Michael's anorectal exam reveals a symmetrical zone of redness around the anus. The skin has ridges and there are superficial erosions. There are small skin tags. Tone and squeeze are normal. Proctoscopy to 14 cm reveals grade I internal hemorrhoids and nothing else.

Believe it or not, anal itch is a very challenging and relatively common complaint. Most surgeons find it difficult to treat. Our dermatology colleagues, when we can find one willing to see these patients, probably do a little bit better.

I don't mean to pick on Dermatologists. Even some of my General and Colorectal Surgery colleagues will try to avoid seeing patients whose chief complaint is an *itchy bum*. And some Family Doctors won't even examine the anus; they just refer a patient with anal complaints to someone like me.

Surgeons like to provide operative solutions to problems, and patients with an itchy bum almost never need operative management. Of course, the reluctance for clinicians to see patients because their problem is challenging, uninteresting, or is unlikely to lead to an operative fix is wrong. I get upset with my colleagues who try to cherry-pick referrals, seeing only the problems that interest them. This tendency is not that rare when it comes to anal complaints.

An additional and more shameful explanation for surgeons declining referrals of patients with anal complaints is that operations for anal diseases pay much less than the bigger, sexier, abdomino-pelvic operations. This makes no sense to me. But don't seek to understand physician remuneration in the Canadian Health Care system. I gave up years ago.

Anal itch is such a difficult problem that my senior mentor at the

Lahey Clinic advised me to never give a presentation on the topic lest I get a reputation as *the anal itch expert* ... a reputation that would make me the consultant of choice. He was only half joking. As fate would have it, my first invitation to a surgical meeting was to give a talk on anal itch. Of course, I said yes.

Itch can be associated with many anal pathologies, but when itch is the dominant symptom, the correct diagnosis is invariably a condition called "Pruritus ani" (PA). Literally, *anal itch*. My surgical forebears must have thought the diagnosis would seem more legitimate if they translated the patient's complaint into Latin.

Pruritus ani is actually two conditions: primary PA and secondary PA. When the chief complaint is itch, 90% of the time we are dealing with primary PA. In primary PA, the itch is not secondary to other pathology – the itch is the disease.

PRIMARY PRURITUS ANI

How can itch be a disease on its own? There are two main theories: hygiene and diet.

Two Contributory Theories

The major theory is that primary PA is a hygiene problem – specifically, a problem of *over*-hygienic behaviour. Over-hygienic behaviour has been called "anal polishing" or "polished anus syndrome." Excessive washing, wiping, and drying may have begun as a response to minor seepage, wetness, or perspiration. Contributing factors include a "deep-set anus," obesity, warm weather, and tight clothes, especially underclothes made of synthetic, non-breathable fabrics. Soaps, astringent wipes, and medicated lotions and potions exacerbate the problem. Over-the-counter preparations or prescriptions that contain steroid, antibiotic, and anesthetic agents are especially problematic. Scratching causes further damage.

The minor theory is that primary PA has a dietary cause. The most notorious dietary trigger is caffeine. Coffee has been called the number one laxative in the world. I have had a few patients for whom cutting back on tea or coffee made a difference, but these were patients who were in the four to six cup per day range. Spicy foods and alcohol are occasional culprits. I've been unimpressed with the role of dietary avoidances as a magic bullet for PA.

The Treatment? A Discussion

Having made the diagnosis, I give patients a talk about primary and secondary PA. Most of the patients have primary PA and I review the management principles related to hygiene and diet. It is a long lecture and I follow it with a pamphlet on PA. The pamphlet reviews the recommendations regarding moisture, hygiene, and diet. I sometimes tell patients with Primary PA what one of my favourite mentors in Toronto used to tell his patients, "Treat your anus like you treat your eyes!" In other words, be gentle. Not a lot of soap. No rubbing or scrubbing.

Treat your anus like you treat your eyes!

Dr. Earl Myers was Toronto's original Rear Admiral. He trained at the University of Minnesota, one of the premiere centres of Colorectal Surgery in the world. By the time I worked with Dr. Myers he was about 70, and by then he had restricted his practice to anal disease. To this day, when it comes to looking after this group of patients, I do things more like Dr. Myers than any other of my mentors. He was a mentor to me in every way. The Dr. Earl Myers lecture is given annually at Toronto's Mount Sinai Hospital, where Dr. Myers spent most of his career. The Mount Sinai Hospital in Toronto is a world-class (and world-famous) centre in Colorectal Surgery, especially in the management of Crohn's disease and ulcerative colitis.

Despite my detailed explanation, patients with primary PA are often disappointed after the consultation with me. There are several reasons for this.

The first is that patients are dubious about the accuracy of the diagnosis. They have usually been told, often over many years and by many doctors, that the problem is hemorrhoids and that the Colorectal Surgeon will deliver a quick fix. Wrong on both counts.

The second is that they feel like I am telling them it's their own fault. They often have a routine of polishing the anus and applying goops, and I tell them that their routines are a contributing factor to, if not the main cause of their problem. And if they are over-weight, I join the list of useless medical professionals who review the benefits of weight loss.

Finally, they are seriously unhappy with me when I tell them that while primary PA is manageable, it usually demands a lifelong effort to keep it in check and that they will not be getting a quick fix, either from an operation or from a new ointment.

As for new ointments, I do occasionally provide a prescription for a short course of a weak hydrocortisone cream. I use this in patients who have a very troublesome itch, especially when trying to get to sleep at night. Although long-term steroid use can damage the skin, a 2-4-week course of 1% hydrocortisone can be helpful in disrupting the *itch-scratch cycle*. For nocturnal scratchers, cotton gloves may help. Some patients will benefit from the same protective barrier paste that we use on babies' bottoms to minimize diaper rash – zinc oxide.

A relatively newer approach is capsaicin ointment. I do not have a lot of experience with this agent, but there have been a number of reports of suppression of itch and burning in a significant number of patients.

As I said, patients may be unhappy with my suggestions, so I am quick to offer a second opinion from Dermatology or from one of my Colorectal Surgery colleagues. Usually, I will make this offer at a follow-up visit in 2-3 months if my approach has been met with limited success.

Michael has the classic history and physical findings of primary pruritus ani (PA). He is providing more clues than usual regarding why he has the problem and how we might help him.

- Michael is obese. Obese people often have a deep-set anus. In addition to weight loss, Michael should wear loose-fitting, cotton underclothes. (I referred him to a weight loss clinic.)
- Michael has been using products that are damaging to the perianal skin. He should stop the ointment immediately.
- Michael is damaging the skin with excessive efforts at hygiene. He needs to back off on the soap and the scrubbing.
- Michael is continent, but he does have a tendency to seepage after BMs. This is hard to explain but is likely related to his tendency toward semi-formed stools. He will

probably benefit from increased stool consistency, that is, more formed stools. This might be achieved simply by reducing or stopping the Metamucil®.

SECONDARY PRURITUS ANI

Secondary PA is a lot easier to treat. These patients have itch that is due to a specific anal or perianal pathology. All of the common anal diseases, like fissure (Chapter 2), hemorrhoids (Chapter 1), fistula (Chapter 4), and incontinence (Chapter 7) may be associated with itch. The perianal skin can also be affected by psoriasis, eczema, contact (allergic) dermatitis, and infections like candida, human papilloma virus (HPV), and other sexually transmitted infections (STIs). The treatment is directed at the underlying problem. Unlike primary PA, cure is expected.

Having said that, patients who have itch in association with anal diseases like hemorrhoids, fissure, and fistula need to be warned that operative correction of the anal pathology may not entirely resolve the itch. The itch may persist because the patient had primary PA in addition to the anal pathology. Hemorrhoids, in particular, are notorious for being innocent bystanders, falsely accused when they have committed no crime.

Discriminating between primary and secondary PA is usually straightforward. The patients with secondary PA, in addition to complaining of itch, have the symptoms and physical findings of the underlying disease. The physical finding in primary PA is a symmetrical, often elliptical, zone of damaged skin around the anus. The damage ranges from slight redness to skin ridges, skin thickening, cracking, erosions, and excoriation.

Can PA be caused by anal cancer? Absolutely. So anal itch is not a frivolous complaint. It deserves careful evaluation. More on anal cancer in Chapter 8.

Michael got the talk, the pamphlet, and a 3-week course of 1% hydrocortisone cream to use before bed at night. At follow-up 3 months later, Michael said, "I'm about 50% improved." The skin looked better. He had not lost any weight but had otherwise followed the recommendations. Michael felt that he was continuing to see improvement, so we agreed that he would follow-up with me as needed.

"I Have a Bump on My Butt that Won't Go Away"

FISTULA

Omar is a 39-year-old who explains that he developed a painful lump on his bum about a year ago. After about three days of worsening pain and increasing swelling, he went to the ER where a doctor "made a cut." Pus drained from the wound and he felt much better, but the wound has been intermittently opening up and draining ever since.

There has been no change in bowel habits. There is no pain or protrusion with defecation. He is continent for stool and gas.

On examination, there is an opening on the left lateral perianal skin. There is some local tenderness and rope-like firmness under the skin leading from the opening toward the anus. Pressure near the opening produces a bead of pus. Digital rectal examination reveals good tone and squeeze with no tenderness. In the posterior midline, a tiny pit can be felt in the middle of the anus. On proctoscopy a tiny opening is suspected at the level of the dentate line at the posterior midline. The examination was otherwise normal.

WHAT IS A FISTULA?

Fistulas are second only to hemorrhoids as the most common anal problem I see in my practice. Anal fistula is not as common as anal fissure, but most anal fissure patients won't be referred to a sub-specialist like me. Most fissure patients will be managed by their Family Doctor or a General Surgeon. However, when it comes to fistulas, General Surgeons are appropriately more selective in what they take on. Fistula management can be challenging and the stakes are high, so General Surgeons, as well as Family Doctors, often direct patients with a presumed fistula to a Colorectal Surgeon.

An anal abscess – a collection of pus in one of the spaces around the anorectum – will usually require operative incision of the skin over the abscess to allow the pus to drain. You will recall from Chapter 2 that abscesses around the anus usually begin as infections of the anal glands located within the anal canal.

For about half the patients, incision and drainage (I&D) is all that's needed. The drainage wound heals within a few weeks. End of story.

Unfortunately, in about half of the patients, a tunnel forms between the *gland of origin* and the drainage site on the skin ... a fistula.

Symptoms of a fistula can be constant or intermittent. The main symptom is discharge of pus from the drainage wound, now referred to as the external opening of the fistula. In some patients, the external opening closes enough that pus does not drain and the abscess recurs. The recurrent abscess may burst (drain) on its own or require repeated I&D procedures.

There are a few patients who are minimally symptomatic from their fistula and who decide to leave it alone. The fistula won't go away, but the potential for getting worse is low, probably 5-10%. Patients ask about the fistula turning cancerous, and the cancer risk is not zero, but it is very close to zero. Cancer in chronic fistulas is more of an issue in patients with anal Crohn's disease, but even in this group the risk is less than 1%.

The vast majority of patients are bothered enough that they want to get the fistula fixed. That means surgery. There is no other curative treatment.

HOW ARE FISTULAS TREATED?

Fistula surgery has two goals that are in direct competition with one another: cure the fistula and preserve continence (see Figure 8). It should surprise no one that most patients value continence over cure.

Fistulotomy

Fistulotomy is a laying open or unroofing of the fistula, turning the tunnel into an open wound. This operation has by far the highest cure rate. Because most fistulas travel through some of the sphincter muscle, unroofing the fistula involves dividing some muscle. Dividing sphincter muscle carries the risk of diminished continence.

Fistula surgery has two goals that are in direct competition with one another: cure the fistula and preserve continence.

Figure 8

Fistula Cure vs. Continence Preservation

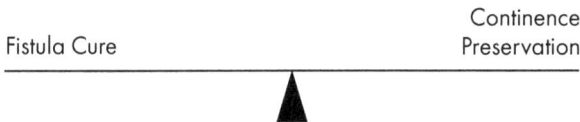

Fistula Cure ——————————————— Continence Preservation

Diminished continence. Interference with control. These are expressions patients will find both scary and useless. Patients want to know exactly what this means. Am I going to be wearing a diaper? Changing my underclothes because of accidents? Unable to work, go out with my friends, play sports, travel? Will I be constantly worrying where the nearest toilet is?

If a Colorectal Surgeon thinks that the answer to any of these questions might be yes, they will not do a fistulotomy. We will try to solve the fistula with one of the operations called "sphincter-sparing" or "sphincter-preserving" procedures. The trouble with these operations is that the cure rates drop from about 95% with fistulotomy to about 50%. There are reports in the surgical literature of higher than 50% success with sphincter-sparing fistula operations, but in the real world, I am convinced that 50% is about right.

Determining Favourability

Since we only do fistulotomy for *favourable* fistulas – that is, where the procedure is not likely to lead to incontinence – the critical step in fistula management is to correctly categorize fistulas as *favourable* or *unfavourable*. Like most things in medicine, whether or not pathology is favourable or unfavourable is determined by a combination of *disease factors* and *patient factors*.

The principal disease factor is the relationship of the fistula to the sphincter muscles. The principal patient factor is the individual patient's underlying risk of incontinence.

Trainees in surgery, called "residents," often ask me how much of the sphincter can be safely divided. My answer is *none*. There is no amount of sphincter division that is entirely safe. In fact, any wound at the anus, even one that does not involve division of sphincter muscle, might heal with sufficient deformity to result in a seepage, wetness, or a hygiene issue. This is rare in the absence of sphincter division, but it is not unheard of.

I think about the determination of favourability in terms of easy decisions and hard decisions. In general, fistulas that cross the sphincters in the lower third (closer to the anal opening) and fistulas that cross the sphincters in the upper third (closer to the rectum) are easy decisions. The former because, in the absence of worrisome patient factors, they are favourable and amenable to fistulotomy. The latter because they are unfavourable and never amenable to fistulotomy. The middle third fistulas are always tough decisions. In this group, patient factors weigh heavily.

Fistulas that go through only the internal sphincter are invariably *low* and can be treated by laying them open. Fistulotomy leaves an open wound that heals over 4-12 weeks. Because the fistula tract is full of bacteria, the wound must be left open. Wound closure would cause an abscess or a spreading bacterial infection. (See Figure 9.)

Figure 9

Fistulotomy

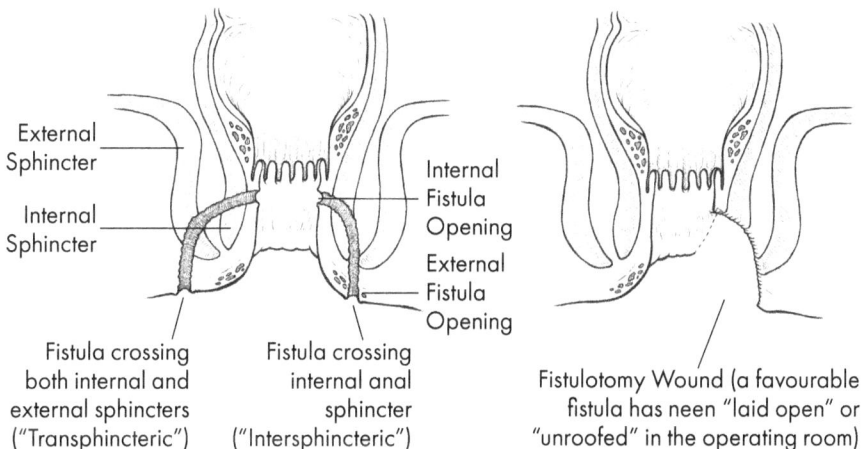

External Sphincter

Internal Sphincter

Internal Fistula Opening

External Fistula Opening

Fistula crossing both internal and external sphincters ("Transphincteric")

Fistula crossing internal anal sphincter ("Intersphincteric")

Fistulotomy Wound (a favourable fistula has neen "laid open" or "unroofed" in the operating room)

Patient factors refer to the individual patient's inherent risk of incontinence. We are not all equal in this regard. A fistula that is deemed to be suitable for fistulotomy in one patient may be deemed to be unsuitable in another.

A patient who already has some incontinence for gas or stool presents us with an easy therapeutic decision: any fistula in this patient is unfavourable and not suitable for fistulotomy. Likewise, a patient who has a tendency to liquid stools, or who describes urgency with the call to stool, will usually fall into the unfavourable category.

Women with fistula can be a challenging group. There are two reasons for this. The first reason is that vaginal delivery can cause sphincter injuries and most of the women who have sustained an obstetrical sphincter injury will not know it; they have no symptoms, they are perfectly continent. But ultrasound examinations of women who have had one vaginal delivery show that sphincter injuries are present in at least 20%. These patients live closer to the edge of incontinence and can be pushed over that edge even by fistulotomy of what appeared to be a favourable fistula.

The second reason that women with fistula can be challenging is that women have a shorter anal canal than men. The front of the anus is particularly shorter. It may appear to the surgeon that only a small amount of muscle is being divided by laying open the fistula, but as a percentage of the muscle that's present, it may be functionally significant. The anterior (towards the vagina) fistula in a woman is one of the most notorious fistulas in the business. It can be wrongly categorized as favourable with unfortunate consequences.

A combination of the patient's history and physical examination will usually allow the fistula to be correctly defined as favourable or unfavourable. This is especially true when the patient's history reveals some urgency, a degree of incontinence, or a history of a traumatic vaginal delivery.

The final decision about whether to do a fistulotomy is made in the operating room (OR).

A Seton

If examination under anesthesia confirms the fistula, and if the anatomy of the fistula is favourable, then in the absence of worrisome patient factors, fistulotomy is done. But if the anatomy is unfavourable, or there are worrisome patient factors, then a seton is placed. (See Figure 10.)

A seton is a strand of material that is looped through the fistula. Most often, the material is a soft rubber, very much like a rubber band. The seton is tied to itself after being passed through the fistula. We pass a seton when we have decided that the fistula is not suitable for fistulotomy because the risk of incontinence is unacceptably high.

Why place a seton? There are a few reasons.

Figure 10

A Seton

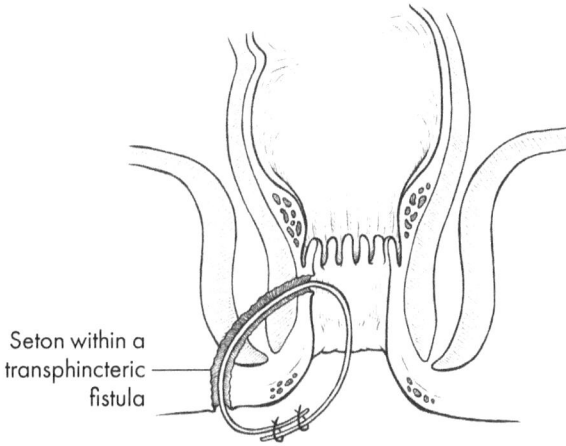

Seton within a
transphincteric
fistula

The seton acts as a drain, making it less likely that abscesses will re-form or that the fistula will develop branches or side-avenues. Also, better drainage is associated with increased comfort, and the soft seton is usually well tolerated. Finally, there is evidence that having a seton in place for a month or two makes it more likely that subsequent sphincter-preserving surgery will be successful. With the seton in place, the tissues become less inflamed, abscess cavities collapse, and the fistula develops more "mature" walls. This, at least, is what we hope will happen after seton placement. It's not always the case.

> *We pass a seton when the fistula is not suitable for fistulotomy because the risk of incontinence is unacceptably high.*

The examination under anesthesia begins with locating the fistula. In addition to inspection and digital palpation, surgeons will try to locate the internal opening by injecting fluid into the external opening while observing where the fluid enters the anal canal. Where the fluid enters is the internal opening of the fistula.

This is a great technique for identifying the internal opening and it has zero risk of injury.

If, before surgery, the surgeon suspects that the internal opening may be hard to find, a pre-operative MRI may be done. MRI will not determine whether the fistula is suitable for fistulotomy, but it is very good at locating the internal opening. I usually get an MRI when the patient's history includes prior unsuccessful efforts by one or more colleagues to find and fix the fistula.

Once the internal opening has been identified, a probe is advanced from the external opening to the internal opening. The relationship of the fistula to the sphincter can then be determined. This relationship, along with knowledge of the patient factors, allows the fistula to be classified as favourable or not. If favourable, the fistula is laid open using an electrocautery device that divides the tissues and seals the blood vessels. If unfavourable, the seton is guided into place and loosely tied.

About 5% of the time, the internal opening from where the fistula arose cannot be found. It is important in these cases that surgeons know when to walk away. If the surgeon is too aggressive in their search for the internal opening, they risk creating a false passage. The patient could end up with the disastrous situation of two internal openings, one due to glandular infection and the other to *surgical misadventure*, also known as "iatrogenic disease," disease caused by the physician.

The plan after seton placement is to return to the OR in 1-3 months to perform one of the sphincter-sparing operations, usually the ligation of the intersphincteric fistula tract (LIFT) or the endoanal advancement flap.

In the LIFT procedure, the surgeon dissects in the intersphincteric plane between the sphincters, the tract is identified in this plane, divided, and then the two ends are tied off (ligated).

In the flap operation, a flap of tissue around the internal opening is dissected and then used as a patch to cover the internal opening.

Both the LIFT and the flap *preserve* the sphincter muscle and have very low risk of interfering with continence. But, as mentioned, success rates are much lower than with fistulotomy, in the range of 50%.

Omar's quality of life was severely affected by the fistula. He was experiencing daily discharge and some discomfort. He was eager to proceed with operative management. Omar had good bowel habits, normal continence, and there was no history of previous anal surgery. In other words, there were no "patient factors."

At examination under anesthesia (EUA), an internal opening was suspected at the dentate line in the posterior midline. Injection of fluid into the external opening confirmed the internal opening. A probe was placed through the fistula. The fistula appeared to be crossing both sphincters at the junction of the lower third and middle thirds of the sphincters. Electrocautery was used to unroof (lay open) the fistula. There were no side avenues. Hemostasis was ensured (no bleeding from the divided tissues).

Omar went home 4 hours later. Omar applied a pad over the wound to protect his clothes and did tub baths 2-3 times per day. He used a gentle laxative and a pain-killer for the first 3 days.

At the 3-week follow-up, Omar was doing well. The wound was clean and healing nicely. He described minimal discomfort and had returned to modified work (fewer hours) 2 weeks after the operation. Continence was unchanged.

At the 6-week follow-up, the wound was almost fully healed. Omar had no complaints. He stopped the tub baths, stopped putting a dressing on the wound, and had returned to full-time work at 4 weeks post-op.

Omar and I were both pleased with his progress. Further follow-up was left on an as needed basis.

5

"My Rectum Is Falling Out!"

RECTAL PROLAPSE

Martina is a 79-year-old woman living in a senior's residence. She is on an anti-hypertensive medication, a cholesterol-lowering agent, and 81 mg of ASA. Her past medical history includes hysterectomy for fibroids, and bladder repair for urinary incontinence. There is no obstetrical history.

Martina has two complaints: she thinks her rectum is falling out, but even worse, she is having daily "accidents" and has to wear a pad. These symptoms have been getting worse over the past 6-12 months.

Martina describes a daily BM, usually formed. She gets an urge to go but there is "almost no warning" and she often does not get to the toilet in time to avoid an accident. When at the toilet she does not strain. There is no pain or blood, but when she wipes, she feels tissue that she needs to push back in. In the past month or two the tissue may even protrude through the anus during her daily walk and it becomes very uncomfortable. She cannot control gas and has daily leakage of mucus onto the pad. She is totally miserable. She has become housebound.

Martina had a colonoscopy at age 70. There was sigmoid

diverticulosis but no other abnormality. Her family history is negative for colorectal cancer.

On examination, Martina's pad is stained with some mucus and feces. Gentle separation of the buttocks causes the anus to open. On straining, the perineum descends more than normal but there is no protrusion of tissue. Proctoscopy shows some redness and edema of the rectal mucosa, but no ulceration or polyp.

Martina was asked to do a "squat and strain test" at the toilet. This test demonstrated a prolapse of the rectum.

Rectal prolapse (RP) patients are among the most unhappy patients we see.

HOW DOES A RECTUM FALL OUT?

The phenomenon is called "intussusception," which in plain English means the inversion of one piece of bowel within another (see Figure 11). In RP, the rectum is inverting, and the inverting rectum descends right through the pelvic floor and anus, reaching the outside world. Internal organs shouldn't do that.

When I explain it to patients, I make a drawing so they can see what's happening. Some patients have said, "It's like turning a sock inside out."

Why does this happen? We are not entirely sure, but age and gender are clearly important factors. The great majority of rectal prolapse patients are women over 70. You would think that pregnancy and vaginal delivery would be major causative factors, but this is not the case. The disease is relatively evenly distributed between nulliparous (no deliveries) and multiparous (more than one delivery) women.

The anatomic findings in the pelvis of patients with rectal prolapse suggest that the normal attachments of the rectum have weakened.

This loss of support is not peculiar to the rectum. The bladder and uterus may have similar issues, and pelvic organ prolapse problems may co-exist.

Figure 11
Rectal Prolapse

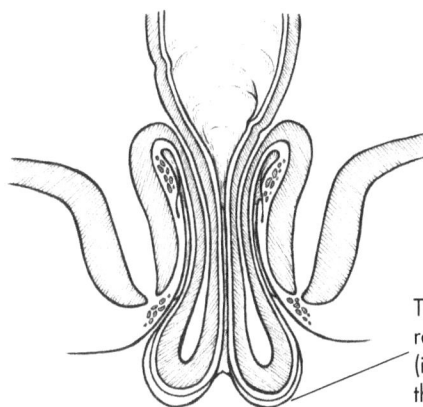

The full thickness of the rectal wall prolapsing (intussuscepting) through the anus

In fact, a problem for women is that the medical profession, male-dominated for most of its history, has divided the pelvis among three separate specialties: Urology, Gynecology, and Colorectal Surgery. In recent years, the three surgical specialties have increasingly worked together in multi-disciplinary pelvic floor clinics to help women with combined problems of *pelvic relaxation.*

When it comes to symptoms, fecal incontinence is often the most distressing one. Patients have a patulous anus, meaning little to no tone or squeeze. The nerves supplying the sphincter and pelvic floor muscles are not firing properly. It is thought that the nerves have suffered a stretch injury. But there is a chicken and egg problem. Is the nerve and muscle failure the cause of pelvic organ prolapse or the result?

There is a chicken and egg problem. Is the nerve and muscle failure the cause of pelvic organ prolapse or the result?

In addition to fecal incontinence, patients with RP may have problems with the evacuation of stool. Again, a chicken and egg issue. In young adults with RP, straining at stool is very often the primary cause of RP. In older patients, the causative role of constipation and difficult evacuation is less clear.

WHAT DO WE DO ABOUT IT?

RP needs operative management. This is probably the only indisputable statement about RP management that I can make. Most Colorectal Surgeons would probably also agree with the statement that operative treatment should be individualized – that is to say, there is no single operation that's best for all patients.

Pre-op investigation is also not standardized. If the patient has not had a colonoscopy in the past 5 years, then I will usually do this to ensure that other colorectal pathology is not missed. But I may forego even this test in some older, frailer patients. I do not do any other investigations.

Although there are many operations for RP, by some counts over a hundred, there are only two approaches to the rectum: from above and from below. In other words, through the abdomen or through the anus. These are formally called "abdominal" and "perineal" repairs.

The abdominal operation incorporates a suspension of the rectum to the sacral bone. A prosthetic mesh material may be used to make the attachment. This operation is called "rectopexy" and it is extremely effective; the risk of recurrent RP is about 5%. Rectopexy operations can be done laparoscopically, that is, using a camera and instruments placed into the abdominal cavity through tiny incisions. This is also called minimally invasive surgery (MIS) and even older, frailer patients can tolerate this approach. Still, rectopexy requires a general anesthetic (GA) and involves some degree of pelvic dissection, where bleeding, infection, and bowel obstruction can result. Also, following anchoring of the rectum, the patient may experience worsening evacuation symptoms.

The most commonly performed perineal operation is called the "Altemeier procedure" or "perineal proctosigmoidectomy." In this operation, under general anesthetic or spinal anesthetic, the rectum is prolapsed and then literally amputated. The non-prolapsing colon is then attached to the anus. I like this operation for frail, elderly patients. It is extremely well tolerated and has a very low complication rate. It does, however, have a significant risk of recurrence, in the range of 10-20%. The prolapse can recur within weeks or after several years.

Another perineal operation, called the "Delorme," is not done as often, but I like this option in young men who have RP. The Delorme involves placing a series of sutures (stitches) in the rectum that, when tied, have the effect of pleating the rectal wall, like closing an open accordion. When used in this subgroup of patients, in whom the RP is often small and the sphincter muscles and pelvic floor relatively preserved, it has a recurrence rate of 20%. These patients are usually *strainers* and they also need pelvic floor physiotherapy and dietary advice. I like this operation for this group because it is almost complication-free, has a very easy recovery, can be done as a day-case (no overnight stay in hospital) and *it keeps me out of the pelvis.* Pelvic surgery in men carries a small risk of injuring nerves that are responsible for sexual function. A disaster, especially in an adolescent.

As with all operations that aim to improve quality of life, it is critical that reasonable expectations are established. Patients having a repair of their rectal prolapse must understand that the operation will not make their weak pelvic floors stronger and that functional disturbances like fecal incontinence and difficult evacuation may not improve. In fact, the likelihood of significant improvement in continence and evacuation are only in the range of 50%.

Martina underwent a perineal proctosigmoidectomy. She had no pre-operative investigations. The operation took 45 minutes. She was discharged home the next day. She had minimal post-operative pain and did not require pain-killers.

Martina followed up with me 3 weeks later. There was no pain, no blood, and no prolapse. She described much less mucous discharge, but there was no change in her continence.

Martina's RP recurred 3 years later. The perineal proctosigmoidectomy was repeated. Martina tolerated the operation well. Five years later there has been no recurrence.

6

"I Have Gas and Stool Coming Through My Vagina"

OBSTETRICAL TRAUMA

Zara is a 29-year-old woman. She had her first child 8 weeks ago. The baby weighed 9 pounds. There was a difficult delivery with vacuum assistance, episiotomy, and a "third-degree tear." The tear was recognized and repaired, but within days Zara noticed decreased control of stool and gas as well as passage of gas and stool through the vagina.

The uncontrolled passage of stool and gas through the anus has stopped, but she continues to pass gas and stool through the vagina. Her family doctor suggested a low-fibre diet to maintain firm stools, and now it is mainly gas that comes into the vagina. She continues to have a vaginal discharge, and vulvar itch and irritation. Symptoms have slowly improved but have not gone away.

Zara had no problems at all prior to the delivery.

I elected not to do an examination at this initial visit. I reviewed the nature of her problem and the treatment options. I explained my rationale for delaying anorectal examination and potential surgery for at least another 3-4 months.

Zara felt that she was coping well enough to accept my recommendation and we agreed to a follow-up visit in 4 months.

Colorectal Surgeons call this "obstetrical trauma." The vagina can tear during delivery, and the tear may extend into and through the anal sphincters. Obstetricians have graded these injuries from one to four. A fourth-degree tear, the worst one, goes through the sphincter muscles and the anorectal lining (mucosa). The injuries are repaired by the obstetrician at the time of the delivery, but sometimes the repairs may break down.

The vagina can tear during delivery, and the tear may extend into and through the anal sphincters.

Depending on the degree of injury, obstetrical trauma can lead to fecal incontinence (FI), anovaginal fistula (AVF), or a combination of the two.

CAUSE AND SYMPTOMS

Fecal incontinence after vaginal delivery is not just the result of tearing the sphincter muscle. Obstetrical FI is also due to weakness of the muscle. Weakness is the result of stretching and tearing of the nerves supplying the muscles. Sphincter disruption and sphincter weakness invariably co-exist.

In the case of a large sphincter injury, the symptoms of FI are present right after delivery, and on physical examination there is a major defect in the sphincter. There may be a complete loss of the perineum – the tissue between the anus and the vagina. The anus and vagina, in other words, become one cavity, or a cavity separated by a thin bridge of skin. This is called a "traumatic cloaca," which refers to a single, common canal for the end of the gastrointestinal tract and vagina. (Like most other mammals, humans normally have cloacas during *early* embryonic development, before the anorectum and genital organs become separate anatomic structures.)

When sphincter weakness is the dominant mechanism leading to FI, patients may not develop symptoms until later in life – usually after menopause. Physical findings are low sphincter resting tone and poor ability to squeeze; there may be a sphincter defect, but rarely a large defect.

Management of AVFs depends on when the patient presents to the surgeon, on the severity of the symptoms, and on the size and location of the fistula. AVFs have a significant "spontaneous" healing rate. It is said to be over 50%. By the time patients are referred to me, the rate of *healing on its own* is no longer that high, but it is high enough that it is prudent to hold off for at least 6 months. As with Zara, I may not even examine the patient during the first few months. Zara's diagnosis of an AVF was clear from her symptoms, and the findings on examination would not have defined or altered the course of treatment.

There is another reason not to proceed with operative repair within the first few months: the tissues aren't ready. Surgeons want some mature scar tissue to work with, and that takes at least 6 months.

The occasional patient is so incapacitated by stool pouring into the vagina that they cannot possibly manage for 6 months. These patients are given a temporary colostomy or ileostomy, that is, a *diverting* stoma. An ileostomy is when the ileum, the last part of the small bowel, is surgically brought out through an opening made in the abdominal wall. A colostomy is the same thing using a piece of colon, usually the sigmoid colon, the segment of colon just above the rectum. Stool is diverted away from the fistula, allowing the patient to cope until the fistula can be repaired. The stoma is closed after successful repair of the fistula. A diverting stoma may increase the success rate of fistula repairs, although this is controversial.

WHEN SURGERY IS REQUIRED

Patients who are not lucky enough to have spontaneous healing of the AVF will need an operation. Very few women with AVF will decide that they can live with it.

The operation I recommend is usually guided by whether I think the problem is only AVF, or AVF along with sphincter disruption and FI.

If the patient does not describe FI, and if the sphincter does not have a major degree of disruption, then I usually recommend an *endoanal advancement flap.* (See Figure 12.) In this operation, a flap of tissue is dissected from the anorectal wall. The flap includes the mucosa (lining of the rectum) and some of the underlying muscle. With the flap dissected, the hole in the wall between the anorectum and vagina is closed with sutures (stitches). The tip of the flap is trimmed away, and then the flap is sewn into position, patching over the suture line where the fistula was.

This operation includes a pre-operative bowel prep (clean out) and a 1-night hospital stay. The post-operative pain is usually very tolerable as most of the operative wound is in tissue that does not have the pain fibres that are located in the body wall. Efforts are made in the weeks after operation to avoid constipation. Bicycle riding and sexual intercourse are avoided for 12 weeks.

Figure 12

Endoanal Advancement Flap

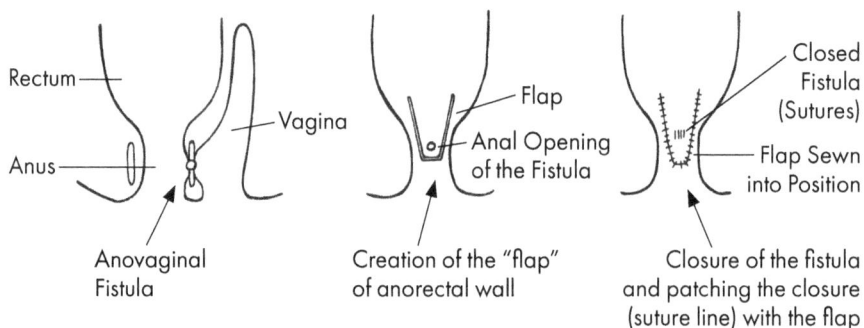

Rectum

Vagina

Anus

Anovaginal Fistula

Flap

Anal Opening of the Fistula

Creation of the "flap" of anorectal wall

Closed Fistula (Sutures)

Flap Sewn into Position

Closure of the fistula and patching the closure (suture line) with the flap

Unfortunately, there is a high failure rate. Just how high the failure rate is depends on who you ask. I think it is in the range of 50%.

Minor degrees of FI can occur after endoanal advancement flap, although the risk is less than 5%. The possibility of needing a temporary stoma to control aggressive post-operative infection or a more active fistula is in the range of 1-2%.

The operation is repeatable, but success rates do not go up with repetition.

Cigarette smoking is an important predictor of failure. Wound healing requires oxygen and smokers deliver less oxygen to their tissues than non-smokers. Patients should stop smoking for a couple of months before the operation.

When the patient has an AVF combined with a sphincter tear and FI, I recommend an *overlapping sphincteroplasty*. (See Figure 13.)

Figure 13

Overlapping Sphincteroplasty

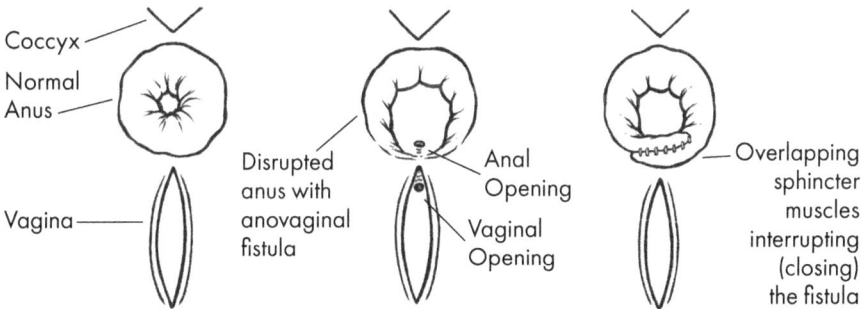

In overlapping sphincteroplasty, an incision is made in the thin perineum between the anus and vagina. Through this incision, the muscle and scar tissue are overlapped and sewn to each other. This re-establishes a ring of sphincter muscle and also eradicates the fistula.

The overlapping sphincteroplasty improves continence in about 70% of patients and cures the AVF in about 80%. Although this is a much higher fistula closure rate than is achieved with the flap procedure, most surgeons do not want to use the sphincteroplasty approach in the absence of a sphincter tear and FI. If the patient is continent and has a relatively intact sphincter, this operation could make things worse.

Also, overlapping sphincteroplasty is followed by a slow and difficult recovery. The perineal wound is notoriously prone to separation. The wound eventually fills in and heals very well, but it can take 12 weeks.

Finally, although improved continence can be expected in about 70% of sphincteroplasty patients, the benefits tend to fade as the years go by. This probably relates to the fact that there is both sphincter disruption and sphincter weakness. Ten years after operating, only about half of patients are still improved.

I mentioned that the size of the fistula can be a determinant of the treatment approach. Almost always, obstetrical fistulas are small, about 1-2 mm in size. Rarely, a patient will have a much larger defect and, in these situations, we use a technique called "gracilis interposition." The gracilis muscle is a long thin muscle located in the inner thigh. The gracilis can be dissected from its normal position and rotated to sit between the anus and vagina to interrupt the fistula. Yes, it's a big operation, usually done with a temporary ileostomy.

The success rate with gracilis interposition is 80%. I have used this technique mainly for recurrent obstetrical AVF as well as for AVF secondary to other kinds of trauma, including operative trauma. I have used the gracilis technique to repair large fistulas between the rectum and the *neo-vagina.*

The neo-vagina is part of gender-affirming surgery. The neo-vagina can be surgically fashioned from the scrotal skin. During the creation of the vagina, the rectal wall can be injured, resulting in the formation of a fistula. The gracilis interposition has successfully eradicated these fistulas.

Zara returned to the clinic in 4 months. Her 6-month-old son was with her, sleeping in his stroller. Zara's husband, Paul, was also present.

Zara has remained on parental leave and has been doing well. The AVF symptoms have improved, but are still bothersome enough that Zara was certain she needed to get it fixed. There was daily gas through the vagina, as well as vaginal discharge and itch. The problem interfered with her sex life.

Zara described continence "on the anal side" with loss of gas and occasionally stool "on the vagina side."

Examination revealed good tone and squeeze of the anal canal, and a slightly thin perineum without major sphincter tear. A 1-2 mm opening could be felt on digital rectal examination and could be seen through a scope (proctoscopy) at the top of the anal canal in the anterior midline. Insufflation of air through the proctoscope could be heard to escape out the vagina.

As with all patients for whom an operation is recommended, I explained and drew pictures of the problem and the operative options. We had an extensive discussion of the rationale, pros and cons, reasonable expectations, potential complications, and failure rates. We reviewed the risks of diminished continence, worsening symptoms, and serious infection that could require creating a temporary stoma. (These are long conversations and it is usually best if the patient is not alone. Follow-up meetings may be needed for patients to decide whether they want to proceed and to feel fully informed.)

Zara had a small AVF. She was continent for stool and had minimal sphincter disruption. I elected to use the endoanal advancement flap approach.

Zara tolerated the procedure well and at her 4-week follow-up she described good continence for stool and gas and no loss of gas through the vagina. She and I were both tremendously relieved.

7

"I Have, Um, Accidents"

FECAL INCONTINENCE

Ann is a 57-year-old woman who came to see me because of increasing problems with getting to the toilet in time to avoid accidents. This problem has been getting worse for about 18 months. She retired from teaching high school 6 months ago partly because of this situation. She hoped to travel in her retirement but it is difficult to leave the house.

Ann describes one or two formed stools per day. She gets an urge to go and there is a sense of urgency. She feels she has about a minute to get to the toilet. When at home she can usually avoid accidents but when she goes out, she wears a pad. She has trouble discriminating gas from stool and has daily incontinence for gas. There is no pain, protrusion or blood. There has been no change in bowel habits. There is minor loss of urine with sneezing, coughing, and laughing.

Ann's past medical history includes two vaginal deliveries 30 and 28 years ago. She describes these deliveries as uncomplicated, but her second son was about 10 pounds and forceps were used.

There was a normal colonoscopy 2 years ago.

On inspection of the anal area, there is a slightly thin perineum, and with straining there is some perineal descent but no prolapse. Digital rectal exam reveals poor tone and poor ability to squeeze, as well as some thinning of the anterior sphincter, but without major disruption. Proctoscopy is normal but insufflation of air produced only a weak "urge to go."

Fecal incontinence (FI) is a big problem. It is common, it has a significant impact on quality of life, and a complete cure is rarely achieved. It is uncertain just how common FI is. It is one of those problems that patients may not complain of or admit to. It probably affects 1-2% of the general population, and about 10-20% of the nursing home population.

DIAGNOSIS – THE CHALLENGE

Surprisingly, FI can be diagnostically challenging. Not everyone who experiences fecal staining of the underclothes has FI and some patients with FI have an underlying pathology that needs to be recognized and treated before the incontinence can be addressed.

FI is a failure of the continence mechanism, an unwanted escape of gas and/or stool. Gas is the ultimate test of the continence mechanism and if a person can discriminate between gas and stool and can defer the passage of gas until a socially acceptable time, then they have an intact continence mechanism.

If you are continent for gas but have staining of the underclothes, then the staining is not primarily due to a failure of continence. It is more likely related to some hemorrhoidal protrusion, or a hygiene issue related to skin tags or ineffective rectal emptying.

Being continent is complex. There is a lot more to it than just the anal sphincter muscles, although these are the most important players.

First, you have to want to be continent. Before toilet training, infants and toddlers have everything they need to be continent except for the will to be continent. They just don't care ... yet. Fortunately, someone will usually be along shortly to clean them up. Sadly, lack of will may affect some of us through neurological disease like dementia or brain injury.

Once the desire to be continent exists, we need a perceptive valve that can be opened and closed by degree, and that can tell us what is going to be released should we decide to open the valve. The anus is such a valve. It is truly an amazing organ!

The internal anal sphincter (IAS) is an involuntary muscle with resting tone, meaning that the IAS maintains a high-pressure zone within the anal canal. We don't have to tell it what to do. In fact, we can't tell it what to do. It has a mind of its own. We go about our daily activities without leaking, and without worrying about leaking, because of this muscle.

When the rectum fills, there is an urge to evacuate as well as a reflexive, transient, minor drop in the tone of the internal sphincter. This slight reduction in IAS tone allows a small volume of rectal content to enter the upper anal canal. This reflex is called the "recto-anal inhibitory reflex" or the "sampling reflex." Numerous specialized nerves in the anus tell us whether the rectum contains gas, liquid, or solid. The nerves sample the rectal contents and we get to decide what we want to do about the urge.

If we want to defer evacuation, we use the external anal sphincter (EAS), a voluntary muscle, to raise pressure in the anal canal until the urge fades. Or we decide to fart or to poop. Our option. Well, it's our option if everything is working as it should.

In addition to the sphincter muscles and their nerves, continence also depends on having a healthy rectum. That means the rectum must have the ability to distend without significantly increasing the pressure pushing down on the anus. A stiff or inflamed rectum, or a rectum with a cancer growing in it, may lose this ability to act as a reservoir.

Other variables in the continence mechanism are stool consistency, stool volume, and the speed of stool delivery. It is not hard to imagine that liquid stool, delivered rapidly and in large volume, could overwhelm an otherwise perfectly good continence mechanism.

So, does Ann have FI and, if so, why?

Ann does have FI and her story and physical findings suggest two potential reasons: a partnership of sphincter disruption and sphincter weakness. Ann's obstetrical history explains both of these factors. A big baby. A long labour. Forceps. That's a lot of stress on the nerves and muscles of the pelvic floor. Damage to the nerves and muscles of the pelvic floor may cause fecal incontinence, urinary incontinence, or both of these problems. This is common.

Ann was not aware that there was a tear to the anal sphincter, but a tear may occur that is not identified by the obstetrician or midwife.

Ann's incontinence developed decades after her vaginal deliveries. This suggests that her sphincter weakness is not only due to obstetrical trauma, but also to the effects of aging. Nerve and muscle function deteriorate with age, and although Ann is not old, the obstetrical trauma pushed her close to the edge; aging and menopause have pushed her over the edge. I am sorry to say that age is the most common risk factor for FI.

That Ann's FI manifested many years after her deliveries also suggests that sphincter weakness is playing a bigger causative role than an obstetrical sphincter tear (disruption).

I am sorry to say that age is the most common risk factor for fecal incontinence (FI).

MANAGING FECAL INCONTINENCE

Figure 14

Managing Fecal Incontinence

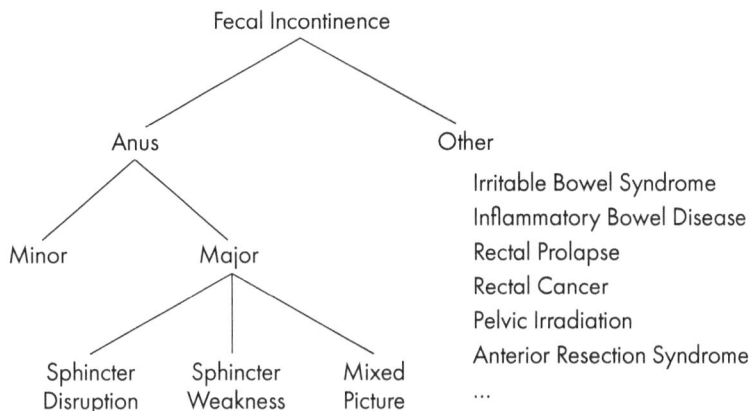

Figure 14 shows my approach to managing FI. The first question I ask myself is whether the problem is primarily with the anus or are there other factors at play.

Patients with rectal prolapse (described in detail in Chapter 5), for instance, are often incontinent, and they do have sphincter weakness, but the therapeutic approach is initially directed at the prolapsing rectum, not the weak sphincter and pelvic floor. Patients with diarrheal illnesses like inflammatory bowel disease (IBD) and irritable bowel syndrome (IBS) may similarly present with FI, but initial therapy is directed at managing the problem of frequent, loose stools (see Chapter 11). Frequent, loose stools that are rapidly delivered to an inflamed rectum might be overwhelming the normal anal sphincters.

A cancer or large polyp in the rectum can interfere with continence.

Pelvic irradiation, often part of the treatment for cervix cancer and prostate cancer, can cause fibrosis or scarring of the rectal wall. The rectum loses some of its ability to act as a reservoir, leading to incontinence.

Loss of reservoir function also results from resection (removal) of part of the rectum. Removal of a part of the rectum is called "anterior resection" and the disturbance of bowel function that results is called the "anterior resection syndrome." Anterior resection syndrome includes irregularity and nocturnal bowel movements, straining, incomplete emptying, and fecal incontinence.

There are also problems that can pose as FI. Grade III and IV hemorrhoids, for instance, can be associated with mucous or fecal staining of the underclothes, but this is not really incontinence. These patients do not describe urgency with the call to stool, nor do they suffer unwanted escape of gas.

If the problem is primarily with the anus, then I try to determine whether this is a minor problem or a major problem. I do not have any hard rules about what makes it a major problem; it's major if the patient says it's major. If they describe restrictions in lifestyle – sports not played, trips not taken, family gatherings missed – then it's clearly a major issue.

REMEDIES

If minor, then the treatment, at least initially, is conservative. Conservative treatment means a bowel management routine and/or pelvic floor physiotherapy.

A bowel management routine strives to achieve two goals: firm stool and an empty rectum. There are two reasons.

1. Firm stools are the easiest to control and the least devastating when there is an accident.
2. An empty rectum can't leak.

How to achieve these goals varies from patient to patient, but common strategies are dietary adjustments and anti-motility (constipating) agents. For some patients, the dietary adjustment is in the direction of more fibre in their diet; for others, less. Some patients may benefit from psyllium (available over-the-counter) to promote a bulkier stool and a more effective rectal evacuation. Slowing transit of stool through the bowel with medications like loperamide (also over-the-counter) can have a significant positive impact on patients with minor degrees of FI. When I suggest loperamide to patients, I frequently get the response, "Oh, I use that when I travel." It is a safe medication and can be used without having to leave the country.

Few patients with minor FI will opt for enemas to achieve complete emptying, but this can be an effective strategy, providing patients with hours or even an entire day of confidence and freedom.

Pelvic floor physiotherapy, Kegel exercises, biofeedback training … the evidence for benefit with these is not perfectly clear. My anecdotal experience working with physiotherapists who are dedicated to helping patients with pelvic floor problems, including fecal and urinary incontinence, is that they are an excellent resource. Plus, like bowel management efforts, physio is risk-free.

The principles of well-formed stools and an empty rectum are applied to all patients with FI, but in the context of major FI, these conservative efforts are unlikely to be sufficient.

When sphincter disruption (a tear) appears to be the dominant mechanism, and the patient feels that FI is having a major impact on their quality of life, then I offer overlapping sphincteroplasty (the details of which are discussed in Chapter 6). The results, unfortunately, are not great. About 70% of patients are significantly improved, but the improvement is not always durable. Ten years after operating, only about half of patients are still continent. Sphincteroplasty is associated with a tough recovery, and with prolonged wound healing of up to 12 weeks.

When sphincter weakness appears to be the main problem, I offer an operation called "sacral neuro-modulation," also called "sacral nerve stimulation" (SNS). Actually, what I offer is a referral to a colleague who does this procedure. I don't. My colleague offers it to patients with FI, UI (urinary incontinence), or mixed incontinence, FI and UI.

After an initial test to establish the likelihood of success, a pacemaker is inserted into the abdominal wall or the lower back. The pacemaker is identical to the one used for rhythm disturbances of the heart. In the case of incontinence, the leads or electrodes (wires carrying the electrical current from the pacemaker) go to the nerves that supply the pelvic floor muscles, including the anal and bladder sphincters. The stimulation of the nerves produces improved continence in about 80% of patients. The procedure is well-tolerated and the complication rate is very low.

Many patients have both sphincter weakness and a sphincter tear. In this group, sacral neuro-modulation is the preferred initial approach. The presence of a tear does not prevent successful SNS, and the SNS procedure is much less of an ordeal than is sphincteroplasty. I mainly use sphincteroplasty when there is a very large sphincter defect. Otherwise, I refer the patients for SNS assessment.

Ann opted for conservative management, including bowel management and pelvic floor physiotherapy. Loperamide proved helpful in achieving the goals of bowel management.

8

"I Think I've Got Warts"

ANOGENITAL WARTS,
HPV, ANAL CANCER

Anil is a 49-year-old man. Over the past 6 months, he has had itch, irritation, and "warts" around the anus. His family doctor gave him a cream called "imiquimod." Anil has been using this for the past 8 weeks, but there has been only slight improvement.

Anil is HIV positive and on anti-viral therapy. His viral load is undetectable and his CD4 count is 423. (A viral load of zero and a CD4 count over 200 are both excellent and are routinely seen in HIV positive people on anti-retroviral therapy.) He has no other health issues and takes no other medications.

Anil has had a sexually transmitted infection (STI) in the past. Two years ago, he was treated for gonococcal proctitis and pharyngitis (inflammation of the rectum and throat secondary to infection with the sexually transmitted bacteria called "gonococcus," which is responsible for gonorrhoea). Because of the "warts," his family doctor did a work-up for STIs, including tests for syphilis, gonorrhoea, and chlamydia. These were all negative.

On examination, there are multiple deposits of warts on the perianal skin (skin around the anus) as well as some warts within the anal canal, on the anoderm, which is the skin of the anus below the dentate line. There are no genital warts. The examination is otherwise normal.

WARTS, HPV, AND CANCER

Anogenital warts, also called "condyloma," are caused by HPV, the human papilloma virus. There are many variants of this virus, and some of them cause not only warts, but also cervical cancer and anal cancer. Unfortunately, the viral variants tend to travel in packs.

Because the variants that cause warts and cancer are travelling companions, patients with warts must be approached with the apprehension that ominous disease is lurking. Warts can produce very bothersome symptoms, but anal and cervical cancer are potentially fatal illnesses. I manage female patients with anal HPV infection in collaboration with my Gynecology colleagues because of the cervical cancer threat.

Disclaimer: Most Colorectal Surgeons, including me, are not HPV experts.

HPV is a sexually transmitted infection (STI) and I frequently consult with my Infectious Disease (ID) colleagues who are more knowledgeable than I about STIs. Patients with warts may need management of gonorrhoea, syphilis, herpes, chlamydia, and/or HIV, and ID specialists are much more proficient in the work-up and treatment of these infections.

So, before I go any further, a disclaimer. Most Colorectal Surgeons, including me, are not HPV experts.

Patients have many questions about warts.

FREQUENTLY ASKED QUESTIONS

Anil asked me: How did I get this? Did I get it from having sex with an infected person? Is it from anal intercourse? Did I get this from my current partner? Will I infect others? How do I get rid of the warts? Will they come back? Is there a cancer risk? What about that vaccine I hear about?

I'll take these one at a time.

How did I get this?

HPV transmission is exclusively by skin-to-skin contact. It doesn't have to be sexual intercourse, but who are we kidding. The viruses that make up the HPV family like to find a home in the anogenital region. The virus is not transmitted by a handshake.

Did I get this from having sex with an infected person?

Yes. It can be from a single sexual encounter or from a single sexual partner.

Is it from anal intercourse?

Commonly, but not necessarily. Transmission is not only through anal intercourse.

Did I get HPV from my partner?

This is a tough one. If the patient has not had sex with anyone other than their current partner in the past 6 months, then the answer is yes, they got it from their current partner. Their partner may be completely unaware that they are infected as people can have HPV without ever having symptoms.

Can I infect others?

Yes. Using a condom greatly reduces the risk of transmission but does not eradicate it.

How do I get rid of the warts?

This is where I come in.

If there are just a few warts on the skin around the anus, they can be destroyed with liquid nitrogen or by the application of an ointment called "podophyllin." Imiquimod is an ointment that can be applied to boost local immunity and leads to eradication or reduction of the warts. These options are reasonable when there are not a lot of warts and when the warts are exclusively on the perianal skin. These treatments have usually been applied by the time the patient gets to me.

When warts are extensive or extend into the anal canal, which they frequently do, ointments and liquid nitrogen don't work. It is necessary to go to the operating room (OR). In the OR, under general anesthesia, I do a combination of excision and destruction. Destruction can be achieved with electrocautery or laser. I always do some excision in order to get specimens for the pathologist.

The pathologist may report only warts (condyloma accuminata) or may report precancerous change. Precancerous change, called "squamous intraepithelial lesion" (SIL), is common. Patients with SIL need surveillance. SIL will progress to cancer in about 10% of patients.

Surveillance is especially important in HIV positive patients, as well as patients who have ano-receptive intercourse. These patients have a higher risk of SIL progression to anal cancer, in the range of 25%. Immunosuppressed individuals, like transplant recipients, are also at increased risk of HPV infection and its complications.

For surveillance, I refer patients with SIL to a clinic that offers high resolution anoscopy (HRA). HRA was adapted from Gynecologists who use a magnified inspection of the cervix, called "colposcopy," to look for and destroy pre-cancerous tissue. Essentially, HRA is colposcopy of the anus. It facilitates the early identification and destruction of SIL.

Will they come back?

Unfortunately, after excision-destruction procedures, the risk of recurrence is in the range of 20-30%. The virus can sleep in the tissues for months, so even after meticulous eradication of all visible warts, there may not have been complete eradication of the invisible virus. Treatment will need to be repeated.

Is there cancer?

Unfortunately, some patients present with warts complicated by cancer or with cancer alone. These cancers are called "anal squamous cell carcinomas" (A-SCC) and almost all are caused by HPV infection.

Figure 15

Anal Canal and Anal Margin

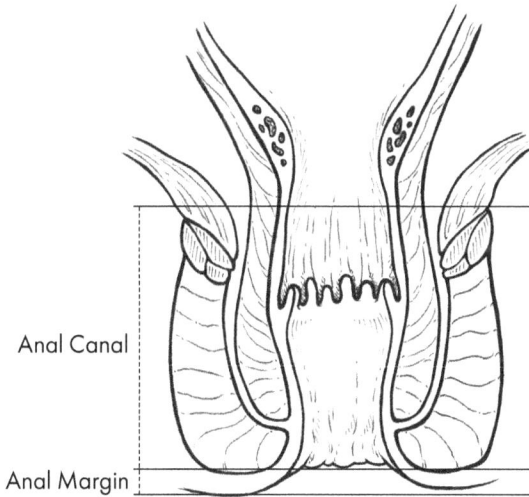

Anal Canal

Anal Margin

Anal cancer may be located within the anal canal or in the anal margin, which is a 5-cm zone of perianal skin around the anus (see Figure 15). Cancer and SIL may present as itch and irritation but are distinguishable from primary pruritus ani (PA) (see Chapter 3) because anal cancer does not produce a symmetrical change in the skin like PA does. Any asymmetrical skin change should raise suspicion, especially if there is associated nodular thickening or ulceration, an open wound or break in the skin. The lesion (area of abnormality) should be biopsied. This is usually done under local anesthesia in the clinic.

The treatment of cancer depends on the *stage* and *location* of the cancer.

Staging refers to how advanced the cancer is. The staging system for anal cancer is used for many cancers and is called the "Tumor, Node, Metastasis" (TNM) staging system. The T stage is determined by the size of the tumor and how far the tumor invades (burrows into) the tissues; the N stage refers to whether there has been spread to the *regional* lymph nodes (in the case of anal cancer, these are nodes in the groin and in the pelvis); the M stage refers to whether there has been spread to distant organs, like the liver or lungs.

The stage of the cancer is determined through physical examination, CT scan of the pelvis, abdomen and chest, and MRI of the pelvis. Fortunately, with anal cancer, metastatic spread to other organs is uncommon.

After staging investigations, patients are reviewed at a weekly conference called the "Multi-disciplinary Cancer Conference" (MCC) or Tumor Board. The usual disciplines are, in no particular order, Colorectal Surgeons, Surgical Oncologists, Radiation Oncologists, Medical Oncologists, Pathologists, Medical Imaging Specialists, and a patient navigator. Management recommendations, including investigations, treatments, and follow-up programs, are made by the tumor board.

An over-simplification of A-SCC management is described below.

- If it's located within the anal canal, it will be treated with a combination of chemotherapy and radiation therapy. The radiation *field* includes the anal canal and the regional lymph nodes located around the rectum, on the side walls of the pelvis, and in the inguinal (groin) region.

- If the cancer is located on the perianal skin, it is treated by excision (surgical removal), unless it is too large to achieve a complete excision, in which case this is also treated with combination chemo-radiotherapy.

The cure rates are in the range of 80% overall, and much higher in the early stages of the disease.

What about that vaccine I hear about?

It is anticipated that HPV vaccines will have a huge impact on HPV infection, especially anal and cervical SIL and SCC. Currently, this vaccine is offered to adolescents, preferably before they are sexually active. The data on its effectiveness in preventing cancer are still accumulating.

Anil was taken to the OR for examination under anesthesia (EUA) and treatment of the warts. The EUA included high resolution anoscopy (HRA). There were deposits of warts on the perianal skin and in the anal canal. These deposits were eradicated with a combination of excision and destruction.

Anil went home later the same day. There was significant pain for a few days but Anil was doing well at his follow-up visit 2 weeks later. The wounds were healing well.

Pathologic examination of the tissue specimens revealed condyloma with SIL. There was no cancer. The pathology was reviewed with Anil. I explained the rationale for surveillance with HRA (high resolution anoscopy) and I referred Anil to the HRA clinic for follow-up.

"Something's Stuck Up There"

SOCIAL INJURIES OF THE RECTUM

Jacy is a 41-year-old man. He came to the emergency room (ER) with the complaint that there was something stuck in his rectum. Thirty-six hours earlier, he placed a billiard ball in his rectum and has been unable to get it out. He is very uncomfortable but not in pain. A plain x-ray of the abdomen shows the ball in the rectum. There is no clinical or radiologic evidence of rectal perforation.

"Do you ever have to remove things that get stuck up there?"

"What have you had to remove?"

I get these questions surprisingly often when people discover what I do for a living. An object stuck in the rectum generates a level of curiosity, prurient interest, and licentious humour that is out of keeping with its frequency as a clinical problem.

NO LAUGHING MATTER

We all understand why, so let's get this out in the open: the anus is, for many people all over the world, an organ of sexual gratification.

An organ of sexual gratification. What a spectacular turn of phrase that is. I stole it from an article I read during my residency and I regret that I cannot provide attribution.

I file clinical problems that result from anal sex or auto-erotic activity under *Social Injuries of the Rectum.* Another great turn of phrase. Also stolen. "Social Injuries of the Rectum" is the title of a 1977 article I read during my surgical training. The senior author of the paper, Norman Sohn, trained at my *alma mater*, the Lahey Clinic, about a decade before me. Dr. Sohn's article was specifically about injuries caused by the insertion of a clenched fist into the rectum. These injuries are extreme, often requiring surgery to repair tears of the anal sphincters and perforations of the rectum. Fortunately, I have only had to deal with a few *fisting* injuries.

Let's get something else out in the open: a cucumber stuck in the rectum strikes us as funny. And I am not going to pretend to be such a perfectly focused physician that I can't see the dark humour in the situation.

"How do you keep a straight face?" Another question I am asked. No problem at all. There are a few reasons.

First, I am very sympathetic to the situation these patients find themselves in. Can you imagine the level of embarrassment and humiliation associated with this problem? These patients have often suffered for days before summoning the nerve to seek help. There is also considerable fear and discomfort. You don't need more than an ordinary level of compassion to take these people seriously.

Second, removal of objects can turn out to be quite challenging. I may even have to do a laparotomy, surgically entering the abdomen to access the rectum and remove the object.

Finally, I have no trouble maintaining a non-judgmental attitude about the situation. Who am I to render a moral judgment? Not my department. I am there to help. A censorious attitude and a humorous tone won't help, and it would be cruel.

"What do you say to some preposterous explanation for how the cucumber came to its final resting place?"

I just say, "That can happen."

The truth is, I have never said that. Patients don't offer an explanation for a cucumber in the rectum. They know we know how the cucumber got there. Still, fanciful stories about slipping in the kitchen while putting away the groceries ... in the nude ... are an easy giggle.

REMOVAL REQUIRES IMAGINATION

There has been a lot written about techniques to retrieve objects. The essential operative skill is imagination. The retrieval methods have to vary with the shape, size, consistency, and position of the object.

I have removed spherical objects with obstetrical forceps. I have removed vegetables by impaling them on instruments. I have had the smallest hand in the department go up the rectum to grab a smooth object. This method was particularly helpful when I was removing a deodorant spray can. I was able to get the can out of the rectum, but the domed

For retrieval, the essential operative skill is imagination.

cap of the can popped off and got left behind. The tiny hand of a colleague saved the day – actually, the middle of the night.

Another trick is to have a member of the team press on the lower left abdomen. Passing a catheter (a rubber tube, open at the tip) alongside the object and blowing in some air can help to break the vacuum seal that holds the object in place.

Rarely, it is necessary to open the abdomen, either to directly massage the object through the anus, or to make an opening in the colon in order to get it out.

When the foreign body has been successfully removed through the anus, before leaving the operating room (OR), it is critical to look in with a scope to ensure that the extraction effort did not perforate the rectum. A post-op x-ray is also needed to confirm an intact rectum.

I have never perforated the bowel in trying to remove an object, but this can happen. I have had to remove glass and clay objects with tremendous care. These objects threaten to injure the surgical team as well as the patient.

An apocryphal tale is about a young man who presents to the emergency room with a vibrator in the rectum. When told that he has to go to the OR to have it removed, the young man explains that there's been a misunderstanding, "I don't want it removed! I just want the batteries changed!" Like I said, licentious humour at best.

A true tale is about a 19-year-old gentleman who was taken to the OR by my senior resident and me to remove a zucchini that was stuck in his rectum. I was the junior resident at the time. The procedure went well. As we were leaving the OR, we were approached by a woman who identified herself as our patient's mother. She asked us why her son had needed surgery and what we found. My unprepared senior resident told her that a zucchini had caused an obstruction in the bowel. "Oh," she said, "I thought it must be something he ate!"

While it is relatively uncommon, there are actually repeat offenders. These patients are referred for psychiatric assessment.

Jacy was taken to the OR. While he was under general anesthesia, a member of my team pushed in the left lower quadrant of the abdomen. This delivered the billiard ball to the top of the anus. A catheter was slid past the ball and some air was injected into the rectum. The anus was gently digitally dilated and small obstetrical forceps were positioned around the ball that was then delivered like a baby's head, with equal care and almost as much satisfaction. Sigmoidoscopy and abdominal x-ray confirmed an intact rectum. Jacy went home a few hours later. He did not show up for his follow-up appointment later that week.

"I Am Always Constipated"

CONSTIPATION

Layla is a 24-year-old woman who came to see me, having experienced years of difficulty moving her bowels. Layla can't remember a time when this was not a problem for her. She recalls that as a child her mother had to give her laxatives, and she has had to use some form of laxative her whole life.

The problem is getting worse. Her current routine is to take two sachets of Pico-Salax® every 2 weeks. The Pico-Salax® gives her diarrhea. She gets the urge to go. The stool is loose and evacuation does not require a lot of straining. This "cleans me out, but it takes almost all day to feel that I have emptied." In the days before she does her clean-out, Layla feels bloated and has abdominal pain. She does not describe any incontinence or urgency.

Over the years, Layla has seen Paediatricians and Gastroenterologists. She has had extensive investigations. She was referred to me to see if there was a role for operation in the management of her constipation.

Layla feels that the problem is "ruining my life."

Constipation is Enemy Number One of anal health. Whether the problem is hard, infrequent stools or straining at evacuation, constipation increases the wear and tear on the anus, as well as on the pelvic floor.

To talk about constipation, we have to talk about poop.

HOW IT'S SUPPOSED TO WORK

Stool is mostly water, and the volume of water in stool is related to the amount of water and fibre in the diet, and to the rate at which stool travels through the large bowel – the colon. The colon's physiologic roles are to deliver stool to the rectum and to absorb water, turning the watery waste that enters from the small intestine (500-1,000cc of water/day) into the much less wet stool (about 100cc of water/day) that enters the rectum. If stool moves slowly through the colon, then a dried-out raisin arrives in the rectum.

Dietary fibre plays a critical role. Undigestible fibre is not absorbed in the small intestine. This type of fibre reaches the colon and acts like a magnet for water, resulting in a wetter and bulkier stool. A bulkier stool stimulates stronger colonic contractions. Stronger colonic contractions produce faster transit. Faster transit results in a wetter, softer, bigger stool in the rectum. The bigger, softer stool triggers a stronger urge and an easier evacuation. Magic.

Infrequent BMs, difficulty with evacuation, or hard stools. Patients may use constipation to mean any of these.

How much fibre should we eat? What kind of fibre? Bran cereal? Fruits and veggies? Fibre supplements? How much water? The answers to these questions are like the part of a recipe that says "flavour to taste." The answers are not the same for everyone. I encourage patients to experiment to find what works for them.

Bowel habits are good if bowel movements (BM) are regular and easy. *Regular?* Over 90% of us have between three BMs per day and three BMs per week. *Easy?* Over 90% of us have completed the process within 15 and 90 seconds of taking a seat on the toilet.

Constipation encompasses infrequent BMs, difficulty with evacuation, or hard stools. Patients may use the word to mean any of these.

DIAGNOSING A COMPLEX PROBLEM

Whatever the type of constipation, almost none of these patients need to see a surgeon. They have a problem with the *function* of the colon or rectum. In general, functional problems are not the surgeon's domain. My colleagues in Family Medicine and Gastrointestinal (GI) Medicine investigate and treat these patients.

But there are two features that may warrant referral to a Colorectal Surgeon.

1. New constipation, that is, a change in bowel habits.
2. Chronic, intractable, *life-ruining* constipation that does not respond to non-surgical management.

A change in bowel habits mandates colonoscopy to rule out a *mechanical* lesion (abnormality). Lesions that narrow the channel of the bowel are called strictures. The change resulting from a stricture is usually constipation, but the build-up of stool and gas upstream from a stricture can also lead to irregularity, change in frequency, and explosive BMs.

Surgical resection (removal) of the diseased segment is usually needed. In Western countries, cancer of the colon is the most common and by far the most life-threatening of the stricturing lesions.

Occasionally, a patient with long-standing constipation is referred to me by one of my GI Medicine colleagues. I follow the algorithm in Figure 16.

Figure 16

Constipation and the Surgeon

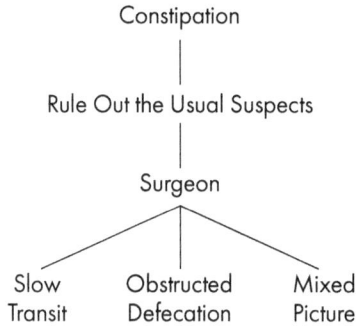

```
                        Constipation
                            |
                Rule Out the Usual Suspects
                            |
                         Surgeon
                   ┌────────┼────────┐
                Slow     Obstructed    Mixed
               Transit   Defecation   Picture
```

Rule out *the usual suspects?* This is a reminder to me that the management of these patients should begin with an assessment by my GI Medicine colleagues. If a Family Doctor refers a patient to me with long-standing constipation, I will usually re-direct the referral to a GI specialist. I defer to their greater expertise in the diagnosis and management of the many causes of constipation: inadequate dietary fibre and fluids, insufficient exercise and activity, medication side effect, irritable bowel syndrome, endocrine diseases like hypothyroidism and hyperparathyroidism, and many other *non-surgical* problems.

My colleagues will invariably colonoscope the patient to rule out a mechanical problem.

GI Medicine experts and Family Doctors sometimes fail to rule out a painful anal lesion as the cause of constipation, but this is understandable. Anal pain is a relatively uncommon explanation for constipation, and, besides, the chief complaint of these patients is invariably not constipation but painful defecation. (I have had a handful of patients over the years who were sent to me to manage their intractable constipation. A careful history disclosed that passing stool was painful. Physical examination confirmed an anal fissure. Management of the fissure cured the painful defecation and the constipation.)

So, I only get involved with patients complaining of constipation after the common causes, *the usual suspects,* have been ruled out and medical management has failed. That means that far less than 1% of patients with long-standing constipation should see someone like me.

These patients have very difficult issues, and what follows is a very simplified discussion of very complex and incompletely understood clinical problems.

For the patient with chronic, intractable constipation who comes to my clinic, I try to figure out if their problem is with the colon, called "slow transit" constipation (also called "colonic inertia"), with the anorectum and pelvic floor, called "obstructive defecation syndrome," or whether there is a *mixed picture* of these two problems. A combination of colonic inertia (CI) and obstructive defecation syndrome (ODS) is relatively common, in some studies accounting for almost half of the patients.

Patients with CI have ineffective motor activity resulting in delayed transit of stool.

In some patients with CI, the motility problem is not restricted to the colon; other parts of the tubular gut, like the stomach and small intestine, may also have ineffective contractions.

To categorize patients as CI, ODS, or mixed picture, the history is extremely helpful. Physical examination less so.

To categorize patients as CI, ODS, or mixed picture, the history is extremely helpful. Physical examination less so.

Patients with CI are typically young women with life-long, life-ruining problems. *Layla has the typical story of CI.* These patients move their bowels about once per month and only after the use of laxatives like PEG (polyethylene glycol) and Pico-Salax®. These young women typically have abdominal pain and bloating in the week or two before defecation. They may even experience nausea and vomiting. They do not typically strain or sit on the toilet for hours.

Patients with ODS are *toilet marathoners.* They may have a daily BM, but trips to the toilet may last an hour and are associated with straining that is often ineffective. These patients may describe a sensation of blockage to the passage of stool and may use manual or digital pressure around or in the anus to assist emptying. They may even extract stool with a finger. They may contort their bodies to try to facilitate emptying. Even passing liquid stool and gas is a problem for most.

Even when the history points strongly to the diagnosis, these patients need investigation. The battery of investigations are the following:

- colon transit test,
- defecogram,
- balloon expulsion test, and
- anal manometry.

A colon transit test is also called "a marker study." The patient swallows 20 markers that look like tiny Cheerios™ and that can be seen on an x-ray. The transit of the markers through the gut is monitored by abdominal x-rays for 5 days. By day 5, individuals with normal function will have no markers visible on the x-ray. But in patients with CI, most of the markers will be seen scattered throughout the colon. Patients with ODS may also have an abnormal transit test, but in these patients the markers have been transported through the colon and have accumulated in the rectum.

A defecogram, believe it or not, is a motion-picture of the defecation process taken with x-ray or MRI. The rectum is filled with a pasty material and then the patient is instructed to evacuate the material while the process is radiologically videoed. Video poop-o-grams need cautious interpretation. Afterall, emptying one's rectum in a radiology suite, in front of doctors and technicians, is not a true simulation of normal defecation. Nonetheless, in patients with ODS, the defecogram will often demonstrate failure of the ano-rectal angle to open, failure of the rectum to empty, and in-folding of the rectal wall (intussusception), which may block the anus and prevent evacuation.

The balloon expulsion test is low-tech and surprisingly discriminating. Normal people who have a 50cc balloon inflated in their rectum get a strong sensation to defecate and can evacuate the balloon in under 60 seconds. Patients with pure CI can also empty the balloon from their rectum. Patients with ODS cannot.

Anal manometry measures intra-anal pressures, both at rest and with squeezing. The ability of the patient to appreciate distention of the rectum, called "rectal sensation," is also tested. Relaxation of the internal anal sphincter in response to rectal distention, *the rectoanal inhibitory reflex,* is identified. These are all expected to be normal in CI, but may be abnormal in patients with ODS.

The history and the four special tests usually allow categorization of these patients as CI, ODS, or mixed picture.

TREATMENT OPTIONS

Treatment options can be recommended as outlined in Figure 17.

For patients who have pure CI, removing the colon and attaching the small bowel to the rectum, can often solve the problem. The operation is called subtotal colectomy with ileorectal anastomosis (STC-IRA). An operation to treat constipation! I know, it sounds drastic. It is drastic. It also remains a bit controversial. It shouldn't be. The science is clear. STC-IRA can greatly improve the quality of life for patients with CI. Of course, the operation is deployed only in patients whose symptoms are both debilitating and unresponsive to all other efforts.

For patients with ODS, the role for operation is more limited. Many of these patients are found on testing to have *dyssynergic defecation.* This is a failure of the pelvic floor muscles to relax during defecation. Non-relaxation of the muscles means that the anorectal angle cannot open and the rectum cannot empty, at least, not easily. One approach to treatment is to re-train the pelvic floor to relax during defecation. Re-training can be achieved with a technique called "biofeedback," or through pelvic floor physiotherapy. These approaches are very helpful, but relapse and re-treatment are common.

Figure 17

Treatment Options

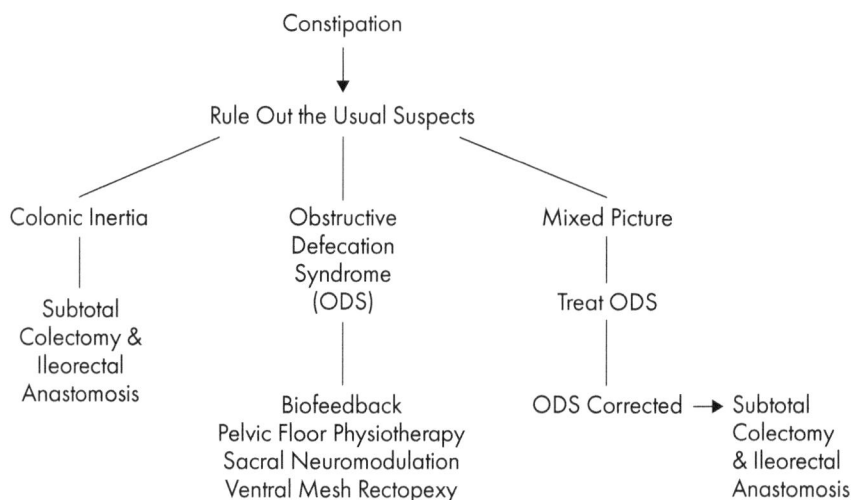

If ODS patients are found to have internal intussusception of the rectum (infolding of the rectal wall) and if biofeedback or physiotherapy are incompletely effective, then consideration can be given to operative management. (See Chapter 5 for a discussion of intussusception of the rectum.) The operation with the best results is the ventral mesh rectopexy (see Figure 18). In this operation a thin sheet of mesh is anchored deep in the pelvis, sewn to the front wall of the rectum, and then anchored to the top of the sacral bone. The mesh prevents the infolding of the rectal wall and alleviates the need to strain.

A lot of Colorectal Surgeons decline to see patients with chronic constipation. The great majority of these patients do not have an operative solution to their problem, and selecting those few patients who might benefit from subtotal colectomy or from ventral mesh rectopexy is extremely challenging. And the results are inconsistent. These patients are best looked after by multi-disciplinary teams that include experts from the worlds of GI Medicine, Biofeedback, Physiotherapy, Psychology, Medical Imaging, Urogynecology, and Colorectal Surgery.

Figure 18

Ventral Mesh Rectopexy

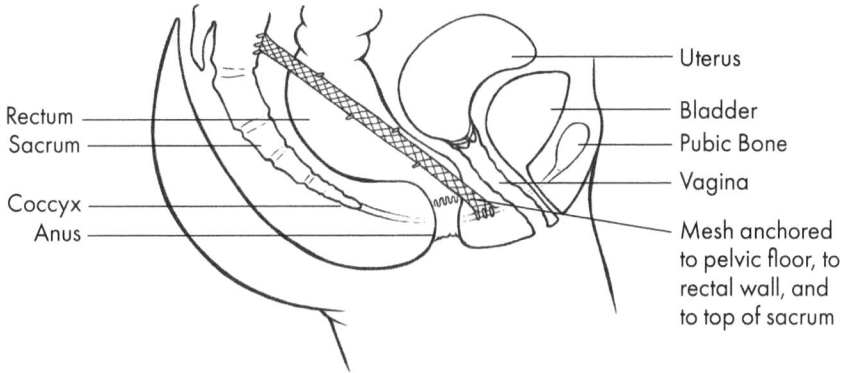

Layla's history suggested that she had CI (or slow transit constipation). She was highly motivated to deal with this and after completing the history and physical examination, I sent her for the four tests. Anal manometry, balloon expulsion, and defecography were all normal. However, the colon transit test demonstrated slow transit.

Layla and I reviewed the diagnosis as well as the option of subtotal colectomy with ileorectal anastomosis. For that follow-up visit to the clinic I had asked Layla if she would like to have a family member or friend accompany her. She brought her mother.

I explained to Layla and her mother the rationale for the operation and the reasonable expectations, as well as the potential complications. About 80% of patients are pleased with the results of the operation. Patients will usually have 4-6 BMs per day. The stool will tend to be semi-formed or liquid. Unfortunately, the symptoms of abdominal discomfort and bloating do not respond as reliably as the constipation, although most patients have less severe complaints.

Layla was completely fed up and elected to proceed with subtotal colectomy and ileorectal anastomosis. She was very pleased with the results.

"I Have Diarrhea and Abdominal Pain"

INFLAMMATORY
BOWEL DISEASE

Jake is a 20-year-old man who was referred to me by his Gastro-enterologist because of medically-intractable ulcerative colitis.

Jake has an 18-month history of frequent loose stools, urgency, and abdominal pain. He was having about 6-10 loose stools during the day and was often awakened from sleep with the need to have a BM. There was often some blood in the stool as well as mucous discharge. He often had a feeling of incomplete emptying after BMs. There was severe lethargy as well as some weight loss.

Jake's symptoms improved with medical therapy, including pred-nisone (a corticosteroid medication that reduces inflammation) and infliximab (a biologic agent that also targets the immune system and reduces inflammation), but whenever he tries to lower the dose of prednisone, his symptoms become intolerable. He is steroid-dependant and the prednisone is causing Jake to have mood swings, weight gain, a moon-shaped face, and muscle weakness. He has had to take a leave from his university studies.

Jake is fed up with the symptoms and the side effects and wants to explore his surgical options.

DISTINGUISHING BETWEEN IBDs

Ulcerative colitis (UC) and Crohn's disease (CD) are chronic, non-infectious inflammations of the gastrointestinal (GI) tract. They are grouped together as inflammatory bowel disease (IBD) because they have so much in common. (See also Figure 19 for a comparison of these two IBDs.)

- They cause many of the same symptoms, most commonly abdominal pain and diarrhea.

- They are initially treated *medically* (non-operatively) and with the same types of medications: immunosuppressives (e.g., steroids and azathioprine), anti-inflammatory products (e.g., ASA), and biologics (e.g., infliximab and adalimumab).

- They are treated surgically when patients are not responding well to medical management or when complications have developed for which there is no satisfactory medical management.

- They are both *idiopathic* diseases, that is, of uncertain cause. It is likely that IBD is the result of an immune response to some environmental trigger in people who are genetically prone to develop these diseases. The diseases in which the immune system attacks parts of our own bodies are called "autoimmune diseases." In both UC and CD patients, the immune system may attack not only the gut, but also the skin, the eyes, and the joints. These are *extra-intestinal manifestations* of IBD.

- They tend to affect young adults, although both diseases can be seen in paediatric and geriatric age groups.

- They are mainly seen in high-income countries, like the US, Canada, Australia, and the UK, although the global distribution is changing with industrialization throughout the world.

There are also important differences.

- The biggest difference between UC and CD is that CD can affect any segment of the gastrointestinal tract, from mouth to anus. UC, on the other hand, is a disease that only affects the colon and rectum. UC always affects the rectum along with a variable amount of the colon, often the entire colon. UC does not affect the anus or the small bowel, while CD very often affects the anus and the small bowel.

- The fact that UC affects only the colon and rectum gives rise to another big difference between UC and CD: curability. UC can be *cured* by surgically removing the diseased organs. Segments of bowel affected by CD can be surgically removed, but the disease usually comes back, recurring at the same site or at other sites in the bowel. In CD, we speak of *control,* not *cure.* (Even in the case of UC we have to be careful with the word "cure." We can cure the colorectal symptoms by surgically removing the colon and rectum. The underlying autoimmune condition is not removed, and some extra-intestinal manifestations may persist. Also, removal of the colon and rectum can produce new problems.)

- In UC, only the inner lining of the colon and rectum, called the "mucosa," is inflamed. In CD, inflammation affects the full thickness of the bowel wall.

The symptoms of mucosal inflammation in patients with UC are loose, frequent, and often bloody bowel movements (BM), abdominal discomfort, bloating, urgency, and feelings of incomplete evacuation. Passage of stool may be accompanied by mucous discharge.

The symptoms of CD depend on which segment of the GI tract is involved. When the colon and rectum are involved, the symptoms are the same as in UC. When the small bowel is involved, the dominant symptom is abdominal pain. CD of the anus has many manifestations ranging from minor skin tags to destructive inflammation and infections.

Figure 19

Ulcerative Colitis (UC) vs. Crohn's Disease (CD)

	Crohn's Disease	Ulcerative Colitis
Parts of Body Affected	Any part of the GI tract (mouth to anus)	Colon and Rectum – not small intestine or anus
Curability	Can be controlled, not cured	Curable
Symptoms	Depending on part of the GI tract affected, includes: abdominal pain, anal skin tags, anal inflammation, anal infections	Loose and frequent bowel movements, sometimes bloody, abdominal discomfort, bloating, urgency, stool with mucus discharge

CURABILITY

A big difference between UC and CD is the potential to cure UC by surgically removing the affected part of the gut. Unlike CD which is characterized by recurrence after bowel resection, UC does not recur after the colon and rectum have been removed. But as we shall see, that does not translate into a *complete* cure of UC.

Ulcerative Colitis (UC)

The surgery for UC is almost always the complete removal of the colon and rectum. By far the most common reason for operative management of UC is *medical intractability.* This means that the symptoms of the disease, or the side effects of the medications used to treat the disease, or a combination of symptoms and side effects are not allowing the patient to have an *adequate* quality of life and an *adequate* quality of health. *This is the situation with Jake.*

Adequate means whatever the patient says it means. And it means different things to different patients. Some patients get fed up with symptoms and medication side effects very quickly and want to explore operative options within months of

> *"Adequate" quality of life and health means whatever the patient says it means.*

diagnosis; other patients try to avoid an operation until it is literally a matter of life and death. About one-third of UC patients ultimately undergo removal of the colon and rectum.

Removal of the colon and rectum in UC patients can be followed either by creation of an ileostomy or by *restoring intestinal continuity,* attaching the small bowel to the anus. When patients select the restorative option, a reservoir or *pouch* is made from the last 40 cm of the small bowel and this *ileal pouch* is attached to the anus. The operation is called "ileal pouch anal anastomosis" (IPAA) (see Figure 20). The most commonly constructed pouch is called a "J-pouch." The pouch is a *neo-rectum,* and provides a reservoir that improves function.

Over 90% of UC patients who elect to proceed with an operation, select the IPAA.

Some patients have such severe attacks of UC that emergency surgery is needed in order to stop bleeding or to prevent imminent colonic perforation. In an emergency situation, the colon is removed and a temporary ileostomy is made. The rectum is left in the pelvis. When the patient has recovered from the acute illness, IPAA may be done.

IPAA restores continuity, preserving the normal route of evacuation through the anus, but the route is really the only thing that's normal. Without a colon to absorb water and without a real rectum, bowel function is good, but it's far from normal. Most patients have about six BMs during day and many have one or two during the night. The stool tends to be loose or semi-formed. Continence is typically excellent during the day, but seepage during sleep may be an issue for some patients.

Figure 20

Ileal Pouch Anal Anastomosis (IPAA)

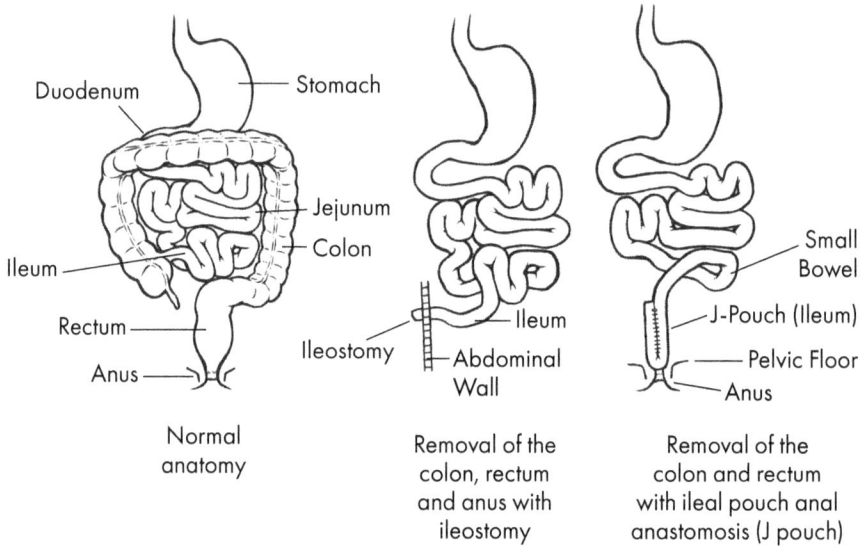

Normal anatomy

Removal of the colon, rectum and anus with ileostomy

Removal of the colon and rectum with ileal pouch anal anastomosis (J pouch)

Many IPAA patients will use anti-diarrheal medications and make dietary adjustments to improve their bowel function.

Complications of IPAA surgery are common, and the failure rate, that is, the need to establish a permanent ileostomy, is about 5%. The most common complication is *pouchitis,* an inflammation of the pouch, probably also an autoimmune phenomenon. Pouchitis usually responds well to medical management, but it can be a chronic, recurrent problem.

There are two complications that deserve special mention: decreased fertility in females and sexual dysfunction in both sexes. Decreased female fertility is related to kinking and blockage of the fallopian tubes by scar tissue. Scarring is a normal consequence of operations. The magnitude of the risk is difficult to define.

Sexual dysfunction in men and women is due to injury to the delicate nerves in the pelvis that supply the organs of sexual function. The risk is small, but the issue is critically important.

Despite the imperfect function and the high rate of complications, IPAA is by far the most common operation performed in UC patients.

Women with IPAA who get pregnant may prefer to deliver by Caesarean section. I endorse this approach. Minor anal sphincter injuries occur in about 20% of women during vaginal delivery. In women with normal anatomy, these injuries rarely cause any incontinence. But in women with IPAA, even minor injuries can cause trouble.

A significant bonus for patients having surgery for UC is cancer prevention. Long-standing UC is associated with an increased risk of colon and rectal cancer. The magnitude of this risk is not very clear and is mainly related to the duration of disease. The risk starts to go up after 8-10 years and continues to rise. The risk is lowered by medical management of UC and by having a colonoscopy at 1-2-year intervals.

Between the extra-intestinal manifestations that may persist, the frequency of pouchitis (in the range of 40%), and the imperfect function of the IPAA, I balk at calling the IPAA "a complete cure" of UC.

Crohn's Disease (CD)

Because CD can affect any part of the gut, the role of surgery is primarily guided by anatomic location. The most common site of CD is the terminal ileum (TI), where the small bowel joins the large bowel. The *transmural* (full thickness of the bowel wall) inflammation of CD produces two types of problems: *obstruction* and *perforation*, and these are not mutually exclusive phenomena.

Obstruction occurs because chronic inflammation thickens the bowel wall and narrows the channel. The narrowing, or stenosis, interferes with the movement of contents through the bowel. Patients experience bloating, cramping, nausea, vomiting, and irregular frequency and consistency of bowel movements. Symptoms are worse after meals and patients may develop food avoidance, *food fear,* and weight loss. When medication does not relieve the symptoms, the obstructing segment is surgically removed.

Perforation occurs when inflammation breaches the wall of the bowel, allowing the gut bacteria to migrate through. Because this tends to be a slow process, the resulting infection is almost always walled off as a collection of pus, an abscess. The abscess may erode into an adjacent structure producing an abnormal connection, a fistula. Abscess and fistula usually lead to surgical resection of the affected segment.

When CD affects only the colon and rectum, it can look so much like UC that it may be indistinguishable. This situation is called indeterminate colitis (IC). Like UC, Crohn's colitis and IC are treated surgically when tolerable medical management has failed. IC patients can have IPAA but suffer higher failure rates than UC patients, about 15% versus 5%. Patients with CD of the colon and rectum who need surgery are not usually offered IPAA because of the higher risk of failure, in the range of 30% or more.

When CD affects only a segment of the colon, removal of the diseased segment is an option.

The anus is an extremely common site of CD. Patients with anal CD usually also have disease at other sites in the GI tract at the same time.

CD can produce anal stenosis, a narrowing of the channel. If severe enough, the patient may be taken to the operating room for anal dilation under anesthesia. This often needs to be repeated at intervals.

A more common and more challenging manifestation of anal CD is abscess-fistula disease. As in patients without CD, the abscess usually arises from infection of an anal gland (see Chapter 2). Spontaneous or operative drainage of the abscess invariably leads to a fistula, a tunnel from the gland of origin to the drainage site (see Chapter 4). Women are at risk of ano-vaginal fistula, a notoriously miserable problem that is very hard to solve (see Chapter 6).

In patients with CD, we rarely perform fistulotomy, the operation where the fistula is unroofed. The anus and surrounding tissues are often chronically inflamed and wounds may not heal. Patients may be bothered as much by the persistent wound as they were by the fistula. Also, fistulas usually travel through some of the sphincter muscle, so laying open of fistulas divides some sphincter. In patients who have a disease associated with loose stools, this can cause incontinence.

It used to be said that more CD patients were made incontinent by surgeons than by their disease. This is no longer true.

Surgeons take a distinctly cautious approach to anal CD. The mantra that we live by is, "Control symptoms, preserve function, do no harm." In the case of abscess-fistula, the management algorithm is: drain the abscess(es), place a seton(s) through the fistula(s) to ensure that drainage is maintained, and then add medical therapy to include a medication like infliximab or adalimumab. The seton(s) is usually removed after a few months. The fistula is not cured but symptom control is almost always achieved.

Colorectal Surgeons live by the mantra, "Control symptoms, preserve function, do no harm."

CD patients are not immune to the same anal diseases as everyone else and may develop painful fissures and symptomatic hemorrhoids. Conservative management is preferred, but if symptoms are not responding to non-operative management, and if the anorectum does not show features of CD, then these patients can have operative treatments like lateral internal sphincterotomy and hemorrhoidectomy (see Chapter 1).

In about 10% of patients with anal involvement, the disease is uncontrollable and unbearable. For those patients, surgical removal of the anus and rectum with colostomy is offered.

If long-standing, UC has a cancer risk, but what about long-standing CD? I'm afraid the answer is yes. The risk is small and hard to quantify, but sites of chronic CD inflammation, including the anus, are at risk of cancer. The cancer risk is not considered high enough to warrant prophylactic removal of the anus or other affected sites, but clinicians need to consider the possibility of cancer when dealing with atypical signs and symptoms in IBD patients.

FEARS AND QUESTIONS

Jake had many questions about having an operation for IBD.

- Will I need a bag?
- Should I take a probiotic?

Will I Need a Bag?

For the great majority of patients needing an operation for IBD, the answer is *no*.

A "bag" is required when a piece of bowel is brought through an opening in the abdominal wall. This is called a "stoma." A colonic stoma is called a "colostomy;" a stoma made from the last part of the small bowel is called an "ileostomy."

The stool that exits through the stoma collects in a bag. The bag adheres to the patient's abdominal wall and collects the stool and gas. No bad smells. The bag is emptied as needed, several times per day for an ileostomy, less often for a colostomy. What comes out through a colostomy is what we would all recognize as stool, with the typical colour and odour, although often semi-formed or soft. The output from an ileostomy is liquid or pasty, green-brown in colour, and has much less odour.

There are many systems for attaching the bag to the abdominal wall. Some bags, also called "pouches," adhere directly to the skin. Some patients prefer a system in which a plate, *the faceplate,* adheres to the abdominal wall and the bag clips on or sticks to the plate. A wide range of stoma appliances is needed because of the wide range of body types, skin types, and stoma output.

There are so many issues and options associated with stomas that stoma care is a well-established specialty called "enterostomal therapy." Registered Nurses do additional training to become certified Enterostomal Therapists, called "ET"s or "Stoma Nurses." ETs are an essential resource for patients and surgeons. They meet with patients pre-operatively to educate them about life with a stoma as well as providing post-operative support. ETs guide the early adjustments in pouching strategies that are invariably needed.

The ETs' pre-operative meetings with the patient include the critically important task of picking the spot on the abdominal wall where the stoma should be placed. ETs and surgeons apply the same rule as real estate agents: location, location, location. There is no more important predictor of a good stoma than a good location on the abdominal wall.

A good location is a flat surface, and the surface should stay flat when the patient sits or bends. If the stoma is placed at the site of a fold in the abdominal wall, the appliance may not maintain a seal and leakage will result. The patient has to be able to see the stoma when standing or sitting. Finding a site on the abdominal wall that has all these features can be challenging, especially in obese patients and patients with scars from previous operations.

The stoma should also be sited so that the bowel comes through the main muscles of the abdominal wall, called the "rectus abdominis" muscles. These are the six-pack muscles more often seen on the cover of *Men's Health* than in surgery clinics. Making the aperture (opening) for the stoma in the rectus abdominis muscles decreases the risk that the aperture will enlarge over time. An enlarged aperture is called a "stomal hernia," and this can produce deformity, pouching problems, and discomfort. It can even lead to bowel obstruction if a loop of bowel gets stuck in the hernia. This can be a surgical emergency.

Stomas may be permanent or temporary. Sometimes they are made with the hope of being temporary but become permanent.

The most common stoma I make is a temporary stoma called a "loop ileostomy" (LI). This is a *diverting* stoma; it is designed to divert the bowel content, preventing it from entering the downstream bowel. The goal is to protect or *de-function*. A temporary LI is most commonly established so that stool will not get to the site of an anastomosis, allowing the anastomosis to heal. This strategy greatly reduces the risk that the patient will get sick from the dreaded complication of anastomotic leak. When surgeons make an anastomosis that has a high risk of anastomotic leak, like the ileal pouch anal anastomosis (IPAA) (see Figure 20), an LI is often made. This allows the IPAA to heal with minimal risk of leak. The LI is closed about 12 weeks later.

Of course, closing the LI is another anastomosis, but this anastomosis has a leak rate in the 1-2% range. It is another operation for the patient, but it is a "small" operation associated with a low rate of serious complications, a 2-3-day hospitalization, and a 2-week recovery. Whether or not to protect an anastomosis with a loop ileostomy requires a careful analysis by the surgeon of the risks and benefits. For anastomoses made to the anus or low rectum, where leak rates may be as high as 10-15%, the analysis usually favours *diversion*.

Should I Take a Probiotic?

IBD patients usually have a team looking after them. The team always includes a Gastrointestinal (GI) Medicine expert, and often includes a Colorectal Surgeon and an Enterostomal Therapist. Dieticians, Psychologists, and Cognitive Behavioural Therapy (CBT) experts, Naturopaths, and Social Workers may also be part of the team.

Probiotics are "live microorganisms which, when administered in adequate amounts, confer a health benefit on the host."

IBD patients become pretty savvy about the roles of the members of the team, and about who knows what. "Should I take a probiotic?" is likely to be fielded by my GI colleagues.

The World Health Organization defines a probiotic as "live microorganisms which, when administered in adequate amounts, confer a health benefit on the host." The bugs of the gut have been implicated in all kinds of human conditions and manipulating gut bacteria by ingesting probiotic preparations is being extensively investigated as a potential therapy for IBD, and other GI and non-GI conditions.

The data on probiotics as a treatment for IBD are evolving rapidly, but at the moment, the evidence is not terribly convincing and probiotics are not routinely recommended. They may be used in patients with recurrent pouchitis, where they have been shown to decrease the rate and severity of recurrent attacks.

Jake and I discussed the options and I answered all of his questions. He left the clinic with some reading material about the IPAA, as well as the name and number of one of my IPAA patients who had agreed to act as a resource for future patients. Jake and I agreed that if he decided to proceed with an operation, he would make a follow-up appointment. I suggested that he bring along a friend or family member to that visit.

Jake returned to the clinic 3 weeks later. His father was with him. Jake's clinical situation was unchanged. He remained fed up with his situation. He had reviewed the material I provided and had spoken with my patient, a young man who had undergone IPAA about 4 years previously. Jake wanted to proceed. The arrangements were made.

Although Jake had been fully investigated in the recent past, including colonoscopy and biopsies, both of which were interpreted as UC, I re-examined Jake's anorectum. Two reasons. First, Jake described excellent continence, but I wanted to assess tone and squeeze. IPAA patients must have excellent pre-operative continence or their post-op continence may be a problem. Second, I wanted to confirm that there were no features of Crohn's disease that had been missed, or that had developed since his last examination by his Gastroenterologist. Anal Crohn's is a complete contra-indication to IPAA. That is, we cannot do IPAA in the setting of a diseased anus.

Jake had IPAA with a protecting loop ileostomy. The ileostomy was closed 12 weeks later, after first examining the pouch anal anastomosis to ensure that it had healed well. Jake's early function was poor, with about ten loose stools per day and about three during the night. He had perfect continence.

Loperamide, an anti-motility medication, was added, and Jake made some adjustments to his diet, and by 12 weeks after ileostomy closure he was having about 6 BMs per day. He was now sleeping without interruption until about 5 a.m. He had stopped all medications other than loperamide. The steroid side effects had all faded. He had returned to university. He and his family were very pleased with his progress.

"Can I Ask You About This?"

The physiology and mechanics of pooping and farting. The pros and cons of washing or wiping. Health issues related to anal sex. The enduring problem of being embarrassed about our bottom-ends. These are some *odds and ends* that demand a little more attention.

POOPING AND FARTING

I talked about *good bowel habits* in Chapter 10, under How It's Supposed to Work, as well as touching on it in a few other places. It means regular and easy passage of stool. Good bowel habits are moderately protective against the wear and tear of defecation. Anal pathology is certainly not restricted to individuals with *bad* bowel habits, but there is an association between constipation, straining, and anal disease. The goal is the Goldilocks of poop: not too hard and not too soft.

The goal is the Goldilocks of poop: not too hard and not too soft.

Let's Talk Pooping

The defecation process should go something like this. We get an urge to go, *a call to stool*. It is generated by the arrival of stool in the rectum. It is not an urgent urge. We don't have to run to the toilet in order to avoid disaster. We can take our time. In fact, we may even defer defecation and the urge will usually pass within minutes. However, not responding to the urge is not a good habit. An important principle for maintaining good bowel habits is *never ignore the call to stool*. Regularly ignoring the call can lead to problems with constipation.

For many patients, the call to stool happens after a meal, usually breakfast. The arrival of food in the stomach stimulates intestinal contractions that deliver colonic content to the rectum. This is the *gastrocolic reflex*. Filling of the rectum generates the urge to poop … or fart.

Why does coffee play a role for so many people?

Something about coffee makes people poop. Not all people, not even a majority of people, but a lot of people do feel the urge to go when they drink coffee. The effect of coffee tends to wane over the years. The effect is seen with regular coffee and may also be seen with decaf, so it's not just the caffeine. Whatever the mechanism, coffee is a strong trigger of the gastrocolic reflex.

What about tea?

Tea is a bit more complex. Herbal teas containing senna or cascara are such strong stimulants that their use should be very limited. These compounds work by promoting colonic contractions. Their effect can be strong enough to cause abdominal discomfort. These teas may be acceptable as an occasional remedy for constipation, but long-term use is strongly discouraged. Senna and cascara can create a lazy, unresponsive bowel, dependent on ever-increasing doses to contract at all. Black tea and other herbal teas are weak colonic stimulants and are safe to use.

Once on the toilet, or squatting in a field, there is a gentle push for a few seconds. Pushing refers to raising intra-abdominal pressure by breathing out against a closed airway (holding your breath) and contracting (squeezing) the muscles of the abdominal wall. The increase in intra-abdominal pressure, combined with contraction of the colorectal wall, moves the stool through the anus and out of the body.

Figure 21

The Anorectal Angle

21A: Levator Muscles Engaged   21B: Levator Muscles Relaxed

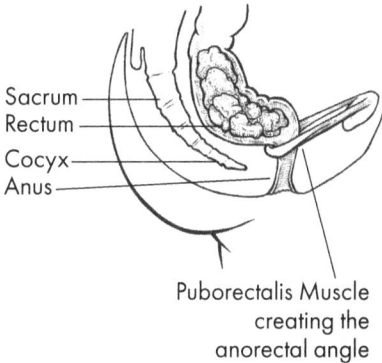

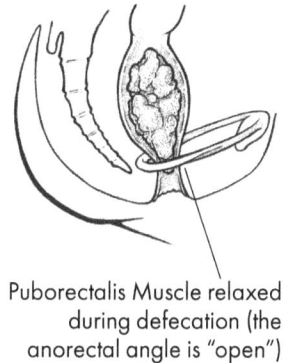

Sacrum
Rectum
Cocyx
Anus

Puborectalis Muscle creating the anorectal angle

Puborectalis Muscle relaxed during defecation (the anorectal angle is "open")

It is essential that the pelvic floor muscles relax during this process. These muscles, called the "levator muscles," create an angle between the anus and the rectum (see Figure 21A). The anorectal angle is an important part of the continence mechanism, keeping stuff in the rectum until such time as is convenient for us. When we sit and gently push, the levator muscles reflexively relax, the anorectal angle opens, and the rectum empties (see Figure 21B). Mission accomplished.

If the muscles don't relax, the angle doesn't open, and mission impossible. Well, mission difficult.

Failure of the muscles to relax is referred to as "dyssynergic defecation." Dyssynergic defecation has a few other names. Decide for yourself if any are of these are more approachable: spastic pelvic floor, non-relaxing puborectalis, paradoxical puborectalis, and anismus. The puborectalis is the U-shaped part of the pelvic floor (levator) muscles and it is most responsible for forming the anorectal angle. The puborectalis muscle must relax for the anorectal angle to open.

Squatting appears to more fully open the anorectal angle than does sitting. This is the concept behind *defecation postural modification devices,* or DPMDs – a sophisticated name for a footstool. The most famous one of these is the Squatty Potty. Studies have shown that DPMDs help patients with evacuation problems. Studies also show that people who have no complaints report faster and more complete evacuation with the use of DPMDs. Societies in which crouching or squatting is the preferred pooping position have a lower incidence of hemorrhoidal disease, diverticulosis, and colorectal cancer than do non-squatting societies. Of course, the demographic differences in these diseases are also linked to other differences, like lower red meat intake, more physical activity, and lower rates of obesity in those same societies.

Straining for more than a few seconds is abnormal, and prolonged, repetitive straining can lead to anal diseases. Straining can also damage the nerves and muscles of the pelvic floor, leading to worsening problems with bowel and urinary function. Repetitive straining can even injure the abdominal wall and contribute to the development of hernias. Hernias are defects that form in the abdominal wall, most commonly in the groin (inguinal region), where there are sites of relative weakness. Hernias form for many reasons, but heavy lifting and repetitive straining top the list.

The need to strain can be a function of stool consistency or firmness. Small, hard, dry stools that look like rabbit-pellets are more difficult to evacuate than large, mushy stools that look like soft-serve ice cream. (Apologies to the ice cream industry ... and to rabbits.)

There's a Scale for Poop?

There are actually classification systems for stool, the most famous being the Bristol Stool Scale™. This scale describes seven types of stools ranging from little, hard pellets at one end to liquid stools at the other. Normal stools are described as soft sausages or snakes, either completely smooth or with some cracks on the surface.

I don't use a stool scale in my practice, preferring to document the patient's description of their stool and their evacuation pattern. My colleagues use these scales primarily for research but some of them use the scales in their clinics, especially as a way to document patient progress.

Poop and pooping tend to disgust us. And the comic idioms for pooping – blast a dookie, pinch a loaf, drop a deuce, lay a brick – do not transform the act of defecation into a charming experience.

Feces, caca, poop, poo, poo-poo, shit, shite, kaka, doo-doo, waste, BM, number 2, crap, dung. A rose by any other name ... What is it? And why the big yuck-factor?

Some feces factoids.

- Seventy-five per cent (75%) of stool is water.
- The main solid components of stool are bacteria, both dead and alive; the rest of the solid *ingredients* are shed cells from the lining of the GI tract and undigestible food.
- The typical brown colour comes from pigments in the bile. Bile is a fluid secreted by the liver into the intestine via the bile ducts; the bile contains substances that aid in the digestion and absorption of nutrients.
- We are genetically hard-wired to be disgusted by stool and to maintain a distance from it. Stool is full of harmful bugs and it is essential to our health to keep it away from where we live and eat.
- Stool smells bad mainly because of sulphur-containing gases like hydrogen sulphide.

... And Farting

Which brings me to intestinal gas, or flatus, along with its delightful euphemisms fart, wind, air biscuit, bottom burp, cut the cheese, let'er rip. Farts are, at the same time, both funny and no laughing matter. Intestinal gas can be a source of significant discomfort.

It is the flammable hydrogen sulphide that provides adolescent boys with the thrill of the flaming fart.

Better to fart and feel the shame
Than hold it in and feel the pain

Of course, as rhymes go, that couplet is not in the same league as this classic.

Beans, beans, the musical fruit
The more you eat the more you toot;
The more you toot the better you feel
So beans, beans for every meal.

Other than one of the greatest words in the English language, what exactly is a fart?

Some fart factoids.

- Farts are normal and are even indicative of a well-functioning gut.
- The main source of the gas that makes up a fart is swallowed air.
- The second source of fart gas is bacterial metabolism. Gut bacteria create gas and consume gas, but the net effect is, you guessed it, gas production.
- The daily volume of flatus is 400 ml to 2,500 ml. This translates into 10-22 toots per day.
- Like stool, farts stink because of their small volume of sulphur-containing molecules. (It is the flammable hydrogen sulphide that provides adolescent boys with the thrill of the flaming fart.) Removing sulphur-containing foods, like beer, and cruciferous vegetables, like broccoli, may help some patients.
- Bacteria mainly make gas from undigested carbohydrates (sugars) that reach the colon, like fructose, found in large volume in soft drinks, and lactose, found in milk products. Beans and other legumes increase bacterial gas production because they contain sugars called "oligosaccharides" that we cannot digest and absorb. Bacteria apparently love them.

- Beano® is a commercially available product that can reduce gas from beans. The pill contains an enzyme that breaks down oligosaccharides so that they get absorbed and don't reach the colonic bacteria.

- Marriage, mysteriously, appears to be a risk factor for flatus. The excellent Canadian comedian Caroline Rhea remarked, "Before we got engaged, he never farted. Now, it's a second language." Anecdotally, I can confirm (from my years of clinical practice!) that marriage does seem to contribute to farting, especially male farting.

The same synergistic events that lead to the passage of stool are called into action for the passage of gas.

Colorectal Surgeons regularly remark on what a magnificent organ the anus is. A mixture of solid, liquid, and gas sits above the anus, and when the pressure rises, the anus can let just the gas escape. Amazing!

Some poor patients with dyssynergic defecation may not only struggle with passage of stool but also with the passage of gas.

WASHING OR WIPING

Wash or wipe? Bidet or toilet paper? I can't provide an evidence-based answer. There are lots of anecdotes and opinions, but there is little science.

Many people, especially those who have multiple bowel movements a day, those who have limited mobility, or those who have a tendency to excessive anal wiping, may favour the bidet as a gentler alternative to toilet paper. Others stick with wiping.

The traditional bidet is a free-standing unit next to the toilet, but there are also "smart" commodes with built-in features of washing and even drying. An economical option for would-be washers is to retro-fit a bidet attachment to a standard toilet. A spray bottle or flexible shower head can accomplish the same thing with even less expense, albeit with less convenience.

For some reason, the bidet is very popular outside North America and not so much within it. It is in 80% of households in Japan, for instance, and almost all Italian homes have at least one. But fewer than 10% of North American homes have a bidet. The prevalence of bidets is on the rise in North America and sales have apparently increased during the COVID-19 pandemic, possibly the result of toilet paper shortages in the pandemic's early days.

Bidets are in 80% of households in Japan and almost all Italian homes, but fewer than 10% of North American homes.

Perhaps the strongest argument for bidets has nothing to do with anal health and hygiene. Toilet paper production destroys millions of trees and uses megalitres of water each year. Toilet paper also has a huge impact on municipal sewers and water-treatment plants. So, in terms of environmental impact, the bidet, which uses comparatively little water, is the clear winner. Bidets equipped with a drying function are especially low impact: not a single square of paper is used.

Nevertheless, there are many among us who stick with toilet paper. It may be because we don't wish to get wet, or because our stools are on the messy side, or it may simply be because we haven't been exposed to bidets and like to go with what we know.

Of course, washing and wiping are not mutually exclusive techniques, and based on my extensive discussions with patients, I am able to report that many bidet devotees are not purists, and take a blended approach: some are washer-wipers and some are wiper-washers.

Wet wipes are yet another strategy, but they are generally not recommended. Medicated wipes are particularly prone to causing irritation, and even plain wipes are associated with polished anus syndrome with resultant itch and irritation (see Chapter 3). Wet wipes are also environmentally unfriendly. Some patients find that a moistened paper towel followed by gentle drying provides the cleansing they need without damaging the perianal skin. (Paper towel should go in the garbage to avoid clogging the plumbing.)

A final word in favour of bidets. One of my colleagues pointed out that if you had poop on your hand, you would wash it off, not wipe it off. Point taken. But I balk a little at the idea that humans should be striving for the same level of hygiene for the anus as for the hand. The hand touches our food, our eyes, and our friends. The anus, not so much. Not a bad rationalization in the wash versus wipe debate. But whether washing, wiping, or a combination approach, excessive cleansing can be harmful to the delicate perianal skin.

ANAL INTERCOURSE

Anal intercourse is not a rare practice. Surveys suggest that a quarter of women have anal intercourse, and about a third of men give and/or receive anal intercourse. And it appears to be increasing in popularity for both.

Believe it or not, I actually don't get a lot of questions about anal sex. Frankly, I am more likely to introduce this topic than the patients are. I may not get asked about anal intercourse because patients are embarrassed, because they figure I won't be very knowledgeable, or because they know more than I do. The last two explanations have some merit. Of course, they may not broach the topic because they have no issues and they're not worried.

Should they be worried?
I don't think they should be worried, but people should be aware of the potential for infection and they should be aware of the ways to protect themselves.

The anus is not self-lubricating and the lining is thin, which is why anal intercourse often produces tears that can lead to infection. Infection from gut bacteria is rare, but infection from sexually transmitted organisms is common. The list of sexually

People should be aware of the potential for infection associated with anal sex and of the ways to protect themselves.

transmitted infections includes chlamydia, gonococcus, syphilis, hepatitis, herpes, HPV, and HIV. For HIV transmission, anal intercourse is the highest risk behaviour.

The risk of transmitting infection can be decreased by using water-based lubricants (to reduce tearing) and by the use of lubricated condoms. The risk of HIV can be further reduced by the use of pre-exposure prophylactic medications, called PrEP.

Does anal intercourse cause fecal incontinence?

It is clear that the vast majority of people who have anal intercourse do not become incontinent. What is less clear is whether or not people who have anal intercourse develop lower anal resting pressures and are affected by minor degrees of incontinence. It appears that anal intercourse has a weak causal relationship with minor incontinence.

Does anal intercourse cause anal diseases?

Anal intercourse does not cause hemorrhoids, but it can occasionally be a significant aggravating factor in patients with hemorrhoidal disease (see Chapter 1). Anal fissure has also been associated with anal intercourse (see Chapter 2). This is important to recognize as these patients may not have the internal anal sphincter hypertonicity of other fissure patients, and may not respond to therapies directed at decreasing sphincter tone. There is a very weak association of anal intercourse with rectal prolapse (see Chapter 5).

Does anal intercourse cause anal cancer?

Sort of. As discussed in Chapter 8, almost all anal cancer is caused by HPV, and HPV infection is dramatically increased in patients who have anal intercourse. The HPV vaccines may have a huge impact on preventing cancers of the anus and cervix.

PATIENT EMBARRASSMENT

"I wish I hadn't delayed coming to see you." As you may imagine, I get this comment all the time.

All too often, embarrassment causes patients to delay an assessment that might not only lead to an improvement in their quality of life, it may even save their life.

Some years ago, one of the colon cancer awareness campaigns used the tagline, "Don't Die of Embarrassment." The phrase is also a popular headline for articles about colon cancer, and was even the title of a memoir on the subject by American actor Barbara Barrie.

It can be tragic when this advice is not followed.

Embarrassment about our rear ends runs deep. Patients aren't just wary of exposing their bottoms; many are too shy to even talk about their bottoms. It's a shame. There are so many words to choose from – ass, arse, butt, buttocks, bum, back-side, back passage, back door, bunghole, booty, bun, caboose, can, cheeks, corn-hole – and we've only reached the letter c! And we haven't reached my personal favourite, *keister*.

> *Don't die of embarrassment. It can be tragic when this advice is not followed.*

Despite this abundance of terms, some patients are actually more comfortable showing me the problem than trying to describe it!

This is an embarrassment we have to get over. To ensure a proper diagnosis, symptoms (the patient's complaints) *and* signs (the physical findings) are required. Show *and* tell. The *history* and the *physical examination* are both fundamental to making the diagnosis, and to developing a plan of investigation that will confirm the diagnosis.

As a Colorectal Surgeon, I am thoroughly aware of these feelings of embarrassment, and I try to make the experience as comfortable as possible. During history taking, I help introduce and normalize the words to describe the problem. During physical examination,

I drape the patient so only the essential part of the body is visible, I explain each step, and I stop if any part of the examination is causing pain. A nurse is present. And of course, all interactions with patients are 100% confidential, and I ensure that all patients understand this.

In the more than 40-plus years that I have been in practice, I don't think I have seen a major decline in the percentage of patients who express embarrassment at having to tell me about their anorectal complaints (or show me their keisters).

"Can That Be Right?"

. . . .

MYTHS DEBUNKED

. . . .

There are lots of myths and misconceptions about our gut. We have touched on some, but there are some that I want to explore further.

1. You should move your bowels every day.
2. Hemorrhoids are painful.
3. Surgical removal is the main treatment of hemorrhoids, and they come back!
4. Colonoscopy is a miserable but necessary experience, and it's dangerous.
5. Colon cancer is a cancer of old age.
6. Colon irrigations (colonics) get rid of toxins.

1. YOU SHOULD MOVE YOUR BOWELS EVERY DAY

Having a daily bowel movement (BM) is the most common pattern of bowel function. Many people have a strong reflex, the *gastrocolic reflex*, that kicks in after breakfast, especially breakfast accompanied by coffee or tea. Food entering the stomach causes colonic contractions that deliver stool to the rectum. Stool entering the rectum generates an urge to go. The urge will fade, but it is best to take advantage of *the call to stool.* Most of us will pass a BM within seconds of taking a seat on the throne, and usually with minimal straining.

Although once a day is the most common pattern, the range of *normal* is generally considered to be between three times per week and three times per day. And most people stay true to their particular pattern, both in terms of the frequency of emptying and the consistency of the stool.

Frequency and consistency of BMs are both prone to fluctuate as a result of dietary and lifestyle changes. Some people notice this more than others but few of us have bowel habits that are impervious to dietary changes. That is why so many of us see a change in bowel habits when we travel. Change may be in the direction of constipation or diarrhea. These changes can result in problems at the bottom end, and I have seen many patients who had their first encounter with anal fissure or hemorrhoidal symptoms following travel-related constipation and straining.

I have even seen patients who became so constipated during travel that they experienced a colonic perforation! That's right, a hard ball of stool, with the delightful name "fecaloma," can actually erode the wall of the bowel. The erosion, called a "stercoral ulcer," can deepen and perforate the wall of the bowel. Stercoral perforation is life-threatening and, luckily, it is rare!

A sustained and unexplained change in bowel habits absolutely warrants investigation.

A transient change in bowel habits related to travel or lifestyle does not warrant any investigation. But a sustained and unexplained change in bowel habits absolutely warrants investigation. The big three symptoms of cancer of the colon and rectum are new abdominal pain, rectal bleeding, and *change in bowel habits.* Colorectal cancer is not the most common cause of any of these symptoms, but it is the diagnosis that must be excluded. The test of choice to exonerate the colon and rectum is a colonoscopy.

See Chapters 10 and 12 for guidance on good bowel habits.

2. HEMORRHOIDS ARE PAINFUL

Hemorrhoidal disease may be the most common cause of anal complaints, but hemorrhoids tend to be blamed for everything that goes wrong in the region. That's not right. Many patients complain, "My hemorrhoids are killing me!" And their hemorrhoids are completely innocent of a capital crime.

Even many doctors refer patients to Colorectal Surgeons with the request, "Please see re: hemorrhoids" when hemorrhoidal disease is not the problem.

All Colorectal Surgeons know to be skeptical when it comes to the diagnosis "hemorrhoids." And fortunately, all doctors, and many patients, know that hemorrhoids should not be casually blamed for rectal bleeding. Rectal bleeding needs to be assessed by history-taking, physical examination, and endoscopic examination of at least the anus and rectum. Often a full endoscopic examination of the colon, a colonoscopy, is indicated.

What is less well understood is that hemorrhoids are not a common cause of pain. The common causes of anal pain are fissure, abscess and a lesion called a thrombosed external hemorrhoid (see Chapter 2). A thrombosed external hemorrhoid is a tender lump at the opening to the anus (the anal verge). The lump appears suddenly, usually after straining at stool or heavy lifting. A small vein at the anal verge has been injured and a clot forms, stretching the tissues and causing pain.

The internal hemorrhoids may cause bright red rectal bleeding. If the internal hemorrhoidal cushions enlarge and the fibres that suspend the cushions in the upper anal canal weaken, the cushions start to descend from the upper anus into the lower anus and even to the outside. This is called protrusion or prolapse of the hemorrhoids.

Protrusion can be uncomfortable. It can be associated with itch and irritation, with wetness and staining, with the need *to push back in* the protruding tissue. But not pain.

Internal hemorrhoids are *internal structures*. Our insides don't have the same type of nerve fibres as our outsides. Evolution has equipped our outsides with exquisitely sensitive nerves that help keep us out of harm's way. Hot, cold, flames, sticks and stones, blades and bullets – they hurt, and we learn to take care. Our insides don't need this kind of information, and our internal organs do not have the equipment to provide the information. Because of this, internal hemorrhoids don't cause pain.

See Chapter 1 for more information regarding the symptoms and treatment of hemorrhoids.

3. SURGICAL REMOVAL IS THE MAIN TREATMENT OF HEMORRHOIDS, AND THEY COME BACK!

While we are on the topic of hemorrhoids, a myth that I can quickly bust is that surgery is the usual treatment. By far the most common treatment of hemorrhoids is reassurance and dietary advice.

Full reassurance may necessitate a colonoscopic examination to ensure that upstream colon or rectal pathology, like polyps and cancer, have been ruled out. But reassuring patients that, "It's just hemorrhoids" can be important. Some patients are terrified that the appearance of some blood means cancer.

> *By far the most common treatment of hemorrhoids is reassurance and dietary advice.*

Almost all patients with grade I internal hemorrhoids (bleeding without protrusion) and most with grade II internal hemorrhoids (protrusion with *spontaneous reduction,* no need for manual reduction, *i.e., to push them back in*) can keep symptoms under control by maintaining bowel habits characterized by the passage of soft stools with minimal straining. This stool pattern can usually be achieved by maintaining sufficient intake of fluid and fibre. An active lifestyle may also be helpful.

Some patients may need a fibre supplement to achieve the goals of regular, soft stool with minimal straining at evacuation. Psyllium and flaxseed can help *normalize* bowel function in patients with either constipation or diarrhea, or both.

Some patients may even need a laxative.

Even patients with grade III hemorrhoids (protrusion requiring manual reduction) may get enough benefit from a bowel management routine that they can avoid an operation.

Patients with grade II disease whose symptoms persist despite good bowel habits, or whose bowels refuse to cooperate, will usually respond well to rubber band ligation. This approach can also be taken with smaller grade III disease.

It is only patients with large grade III internal hemorrhoids and grade IV internal hemorrhoids (chronically prolapsed, will not stay in after manual reduction) or with internal hemorrhoids associated with large skin tags (external hemorrhoids) that end up under the knife.

Hemorrhoids do not come back after surgery, well, not exactly. The hemorrhoids that are removed at hemorrhoidectomy are gone forever. But hemorrhoidal symptoms can recur, or even persist, after surgery.

The reason is that the surgeon did not remove all the hemorrhoidal tissue and this is often appropriate. Excessive removal of tissue lining the anal canal can narrow the canal, making the anus too tight. This is a complication of hemorrhoidectomy called "stenosis." It can be solved, but it is better to prevent it. The preventive strategy is to leave minor hemorrhoidal tissue behind, removing only larger hemorrhoids. As a result of leaving some hemorrhoids behind, patients may complain that, "My hemorrhoids have come back." But this problem affects less than 5% of patients who have undergone hemorrhoidectomy.

See Chapter 1 for a thorough discussion around hemorrhoids, their symptoms, and their treatment.

4. COLONOSCOPY IS A MISERABLE BUT NECESSARY EXPERIENCE, AND IT'S DANGEROUS

Let's look at *miserable* first.

I agree that it's no fun. I have been having colonoscopies every 5 years since I was 45 years old. My excuse for overdoing it is that, if I got colon cancer, I would die of embarrassment long before the cancer got me.

But it's not that bad! It is generally done under sedation which makes the examination completely tolerable in almost 100% of patients. Most patients *sleep* through the procedure. Like most patients, I have been unconscious through all my colonoscopies and remember nothing about them. I wake up completely relaxed and completely comfortable in the recovery area. It's quite a nice feeling! This is the experience for about 99% of patients.

The medications that are given for colonoscopy produce *conscious sedation:* you're asleep but breathing on your own and you can be awakened by voice or touching. Patients receive oxygen by nasal prongs and vital signs (pulse, respiration, blood pressure) are closely monitored.

Like everyone, I hate the prep the day before the colonoscopy. I am not going to get into a debate about the various types of preparation drinks, but my patients use a prep solution called Pico-salax®. This prep does not require drinking a gallon of horrible tasting prep solution. It does require drinking litres of liquid, like electrolyte drinks, also called "sports drinks." But I think there is no question that this is a much easier prep. And it does just as good a job of cleaning out the colon.

There's no way to avoid it. For colonoscopy to be successful the colon has to be empty, and that means several dozen trips to the toilet until just a few drops of clear liquid are being evacuated.

The experience of bowel preparation and colonoscopy have been addressed by several great humorists. I have laughed out loud at some of the articles by the syndicated American humourist Dave Barry. Here are a couple of sample lines.

> [My doctor] showed me a colour diagram of the colon, a lengthy organ that appears to go all over the place, at one point passing briefly through Minneapolis.

> The instructions [for bowel preparation], clearly written by somebody with a great sense of humour, state that after you drink it, "a loose, watery bowel movement may result." This is kind of like saying that after you jump off your roof, you may experience contact with the ground.

Is colonoscopy really *necessary?*

Colonoscopy is absolutely necessary to investigate symptoms that might be the result of disease in the colon, rectum, or terminal ileum (the last bit of the small intestine that empties into the colon). Colonoscopy as a *diagnostic test* is necessary.

Is colonoscopy *necessary* as a *screening* test for colorectal cancer? This is a more difficult question to answer.

Screening means looking for a disease in people who have no complaints with the goal of identifying the disease at a more curable stage, thereby preventing nasty outcomes, especially death.

In many ways, colorectal cancer is ideally suited for screening.

In many ways, colorectal cancer is ideally suited for screening.

1. It is a common and important disease. How common? About one in twenty people in Western countries will get colon cancer by age 75. How important? If not treated, it's 100% fatal, so pretty important.
2. It is preventable. Almost all colorectal cancers arise from a precursor lesion called a "polyp." Identifying and removing

polyps prevents cancer. Polyps are almost always silent, producing no symptoms.

3. It is curable. When colon cancer is found after the investigation of symptoms, the cure rate is in the range of 70%; when it is found in asymptomatic people, the cure rate is over 90%.

4. Polyps and cancer can be found at an asymptomatic stage by screening tests. Removing polyps during screening colonoscopy, called "polypectomy," prevents cancer.

The idea that we should screen the population for colorectal cancer is widely accepted in industrialized nations where the disease is common. For average risk people, screening is recommended between ages 50 (or 45) and 75. Both the age to start and the age to stop are a bit flexible in my opinion. There appear to be increasing rates of colon cancer in people under 50. And many people now maintain excellent health well into their 80s.

I suspect that future screening guidelines will have earlier starting and later stopping ages. Guidelines for screening are published by many agencies, like the Canadian Cancer Society and the U.S. Preventive Services Task Force. The agencies empanel experts to produce evidence-based recommendations or guidelines. As the evidence evolves, the guidelines change.

The idea of colorectal cancer screening may not be controversial, but how best to screen the population is quite controversial.

The optimal screening technique is controversial because colonoscopy is not a perfect screening test. True, it is extremely good at finding polyps and cancers. Almost all the polyps that are found during colonoscopy can be removed through the colonoscope with a wire snare (polypectomy). And, as mentioned, removing polyps prevents cancers and saves lives. Mission accomplished.

But colonoscopy is expensive, and it isn't fun, especially the prep. There is also the significant inconvenience of having to take 1 to 1.5 days off work: half day for the prep and one day for the examination. The examination only takes 15-20 minutes, but because of the sedation, you can't really have a productive work day.

The whole business is sufficiently unpleasant that many members of the population who are offered colonoscopy will say, "No thank you." You can't save lives with a test that people won't take.

Also, colonoscopy is not risk-free. *But is it dangerous?*

The risk of colon perforation is about 1 in 1,200 patients, but it increases to almost 1 in 500 if polyps are removed. The risk of bleeding from a polypectomy wound is about 3 in 500. Perforation will usually require an operation. Bleeding can usually be controlled by re-introducing the colonoscope and applying a clip to the bleeding site. The risk of death is about 1 in 14,000 patients. (Just for reference, the chance of dying from a lightning strike is about one in a million, and the chance of winning most major lotteries is less than one in ten million.)

While the colonoscopy risk numbers are not bad, remember that these are people undergoing *screening*. These individuals had no complaints, were minding their own business, and were subjected to an unpleasant test with a risk of injury and death.

If screening colonoscopy is negative, it is usually repeated at 10-year intervals. If polyps are found at the initial colonoscopy, then the interval between examinations shortens, usually to every 5 years, but the interval will depend on the number and type of polyps. This regimen has been shown to dramatically reduce colon cancer mortality.

You might think 5 years is a long time between colonoscopies in an individual who has been found to be a polyp-grower, but this interval is very safe. The polyp-cancer sequence – that is, the time it takes a polyp-free colon to grow a polyp and for that polyp to become a cancer – is more than 5 years.

The main alternative to screening with colonoscopy is screening with a stool test called FIT, the *fecal immunochemical test*. The FIT looks for invisible traces of human blood in the stool. The test is done at home. FIT testing kits are usually sent to your home or are picked up at your Family Doctor's office. The easiest way to do the test is to poop into a plastic container. Then you dip the testing stick into the poop, put the poopy stick into the test-tube, and then put the test-tube into a plastic bag. The bag is mailed in an envelope to the testing centre. Test results usually arrive at your doctor's office in 1-2 weeks.

The chance of being FIT positive, that is, having a trace of blood in the stool samples, is 10 -15%. A positive test does not mean you have cancer. In fact, the chance that colon cancer is the cause of the positive test is about 4%.

A positive FIT leads to a strong recommendation for a colonoscopy, usually within the next 6 weeks. Polyps, the pre-cancerous growths, are commonly found in FIT positive patients. The polyps are removed and sent to the pathology department for analysis.

FIT testing, usually done annually or every 2 years, followed by colonoscopy of FIT positive people, has been shown to dramatically reduce colon cancer mortality.

Up until now, we have been talking about screening the *average risk individual between the ages of 50 and 75.* Individuals with a first-degree relative (parent or sibling) under the age of 60 with colon cancer, or with two or more second-degree relatives with colon cancer, have roughly twice the risk of colon cancer as the general population (about 1 in 20 by age 75). These individuals are advised to have screening colonoscopy every 5 years starting at age 40, or 10 years younger than the youngest colon cancer patient in the family. These guidelines are usually also applied if the family member(s) diagnosis was a large polyp rather than a cancer.

5. COLON CANCER IS A CANCER OF OLD AGE

I'm sorry to do this to you, but to bust this myth I have to review some stats.

- Colorectal cancer (CRC) is the second leading cause of cancer death in Western countries. Lung cancer is number one.
- Men and women are roughly equally affected by CRC.

- Roughly half of patients diagnosed with CRC are under 65 years of age.
- Roughly one-third of patients diagnosed with CRC are under 55 years of age.
- The rate of CRC is increasing in people under 50.
- The rate of CRC almost doubled between 1995 and 2020 for people under age 55.

Why the rising rates of CRC in younger adults? The likely reason is increasing exposure to known environmental risk factors, like:

- obesity,
- lack of exercise,
- high dietary fat and processed meats,
- low dietary fruits and vegetables,
- alcohol, and
- cigarettes.

The rate of CRC almost doubled between 1995 and 2020 for people under age 55.

Some more stats to digest.

- The cure rate for CRC is over 90% if the cancer has not spread to the nearby lymph nodes. About half of patients are diagnosed at this stage, called stage I or stage II.
- The cure rate for CRC is about 70% if the cancer has spread to the lymph nodes but not to distant organs, like the liver and the lung. About 35% of patients are diagnosed at this stage, called stage III.
- If the cancer has spread to the liver or lungs, the cure rate is only about 15%. About 15% of patients are diagnosed at this stage, stage IV.

6. COLON IRRIGATIONS (COLONICS) GET RID OF TOXINS

Why would I ask someone to put a tube up my rectum to flush out my colon? It sounds unpleasant and potentially dangerous. It also sounds totally unnecessary.

Is it unnecessary?
Absolutely.

Does it improve any aspect of health or quality of life?
There is no evidence whatsoever of any benefits from colon irrigation. There is no poison, toxin, or pathogen (bacteria, fungus, virus) in the colon that needs to be flushed out. In fact, the bacteria that are in the colon are supposed to be there. Mammals have had bacteria living in their colons for millions of years. We have come to rely on the colonic microbiome for some metabolic and infection fighting roles.

> *Mammals have had bacteria living in their colons for millions of years and we rely on the colonic microbiome for some metabolic and infection fighting roles.*

Is it unpleasant?
It is associated with diarrhea and cramps, and occasionally nausea and bloating. So, yes, it's unpleasant.

Is it dangerous?
Not very, but there are reports of infection, rectal perforation, dehydration, and even death.

If you like the medicines you take and the procedures you endure to be evidence-based, then colon irrigation is not for you.

While on the topic of thoroughly unnecessary interventions, what about *anal bleaching?*

The skin around the anus may get darker as the years go by. That's perfectly normal. *Bleaching* refers to lightening the colour of the perianal skin to match the skin of the buttocks. It is not done with bleach. There are topical agents and laser techniques that can achieve the goal. I don't offer this and know little about it. It is primarily offered by Dermatologists and Plastic Surgeons who have a focus on cosmetic therapies.

In the hands of experts, bleaching appears to be safe. I have never been sent a patient with a complication related to bleaching the perianal skin. This may be at least partly because it has not caught on in my jurisdiction. I have to say, I do worry about anything that could damage the perianal skin. Wounds and scarring in this region can have nasty consequences.

Why bleach?

There is no health benefit. The only possible reason is the *cosmetic effect*. I suppose that the cosmetic *benefit* might provide increased sexual confidence. Apparently, it is popular in the pornography industry.

"Do You Like What You Do?"

MY BACK PAGES

A SPECIAL SPECIALTY

Colorectal Surgeons look after patients with diseases of the colon, rectum, and anus ... and diseases of the small intestines, the appendix, and the abdominal wall. Despite the range of our expertise, we are known as Rear Admirals, Arse Angels, and Ass-Men and -Women. One patient walked into my clinic and said, "I hear you're the *anus whisperer.*"

They call me the anus whisperer.

Colon and rectal surgery is one of the oldest and most well-established sub-specialties in the surgical world. We have scientific journals dedicated to the specialty. We have national and international societies. We have scholarly meetings that attract thousands of surgeons from around the world. We have processes for the accreditation of training programs and for the certification of specialists. We have risen to the highest ranks of medical academia. Some of my colleagues are highly accomplished surgeon-scientists.

MARCUS BURNSTEIN   147

Still, by far the most common question I get asked is, "What in God's name made you decide to do this for a living?" It is usually asked by a patient on the procto table undergoing digital rectal or proctoscopic examination – that is, while I have a finger or scope up their backside. Other comments I get during anorectal examinations include, "Geez, take me out to dinner first" and "Tell my wife you didn't find my head up there."

So, what's the answer?

The answer, in part at least, is timing. I trained in General Surgery at the University of Toronto from 1979-1984. General Surgery is a very broad surgical specialty, and it is the point of entry for many subspecialties, like Vascular Surgery (blood vessels), Thoracic Surgery (chest), Breast Surgery, Endocrine Surgery (glands like the adrenal glands and thyroid gland), Transplant Surgery, Surgical Oncology (cancer), Paediatric Surgery, Trauma-Critical Care Surgery, and Colorectal Surgery.

In the early 1980s, surgical techniques for preserving the anus were evolving, and these technically challenging operations, performed almost exclusively by Colorectal Surgeons, were attracting young surgeons. The ileal pouch anal anastomosis (IPAA), discussed in Chapter 11, is an example of a sphincter-preserving operation.

Before the development of these techniques, patients with ulcerative colitis or rectal cancer would have *resection without reconstruction,* that is, removal of the diseased portion of the colon without restoration of continuity. Meaning they would need a permanent colostomy or ileostomy (i.e., a bag attached to the abdominal wall) for the rest of their lives. Stoma means mouth or opening, and as I discussed in Chapter 11 on inflammatory bowel disease, a piece of bowel brought through the abdominal wall is called a stoma. A stoma made from the part of the bowel called the "ileum" is an ileostomy, from the colon, a colostomy.

These new techniques were an improvement. And the ability to provide patients with a restorative procedure for diseases that had traditionally resulted in a permanent stoma was very rewarding, and the surgeons offering these sophisticated reconstructions, only a few in the country, became my heroes and role models.

But mine is not a glamorous specialty. Poop, poo-poo, doo-doo, caca, excrement, feces, shit. Whatever you call it, people have an understandable aversion to stool, and Colorectal Surgery and stool are closely linked in the lay consciousness.

Not only in the lay consciousness. Poop seems to influence the position of the specialty in the professional hierarchy. Colorectal Surgeons know that they peck at a lower order than the courageous Neurosurgeons, the athletic Orthopaedic Surgeons, the sexy Cardiac Surgeons, the elegant Plastic Surgeons, and any other surgical subspecialty you can name. Even Urologists with their pee-pee and Ear, Nose, and Throat doctors with their snot have higher status. The fee schedules in public health systems reflect this hierarchy, which makes no sense.

Colorectal Surgeons bear witness on a daily basis to the fact that few things put you on the sidelines of life more quickly or more completely than a diseased, poorly functioning gut. This is especially true of the terminal 2-4 cm of gut. The anus, when diseased, has a way of hijacking everything you care about, becoming the only thing you can think about, the centre of your universe. Also, many anal operations demand sophisticated decision-making and delicate workmanship. Bad decisions and poor technical performance can have dire and lasting consequences.

Despite the poop factor, not everyone finds what I do to be objectionable. While many people are perplexed and some are mildly disgusted, there are also a lot of people who are interested, even fascinated.

Interest in my world is correlated with age.

The gastrointestinal (GI) tract, like the rest of our parts, goes through a lot of wear and tear. Bits start breaking down, performing poorly, or, even worse, growing things. The anus, in particular, sees a lot of action in the course of a lifetime, and anal diseases are extremely common. Colorectal cancer is also common. It is age-related and preventable. So, among people over 50, the Colorectal Surgeon is a popular and engaging cocktail party guest. Well, we like to think so. (We are less popular at dinner parties.)

Most of us in the Colorectal biz are not much bothered by our social and professional image. Everybody needs us, and loves us, at some point in their life. We unapologetically say that, "We get everyone *in the end.*"

THE SURGICAL EGO

The Pope has died, and when he arrives in heaven he is warmly greeted by St. Peter. After some small talk, St. Peter takes the pontiff on a heavenly tour, during which they stop by the cafeteria for lunch. The Pope gets in the queue with St. Peter and is delighted to see that there is no preferential treatment, that everyone is regarded equally in heaven and has to wait their turn.

But as the Pope and St. Peter are moving along in the line like everybody else, a white-haired, white-bearded man in a green surgical scrub suit and white lab coat rushes past to the head of the line, grabs his lunch and hurries off. The Pope is taken aback. "Who was that?" he asks. St. Peter explains, "Oh, that's God. He likes to pretend he's a surgeon."

This joke, one of my favourite doctor jokes, reflects the common perception of surgeons as self-important and egotistical. Here's another one.

A pathologist, an internal medicine specialist, and a surgeon have gone duck hunting. As they hide in a field, a large bird flies overhead, and the internal medicine specialist, looking through his high-powered binoculars, begins a detailed description. He starts to list the various types of bird it could be. "Is it a mallard duck? It could be a loon? Maybe it's a goose or an eagle?" While this is going on, the surgeon takes aim, shoots the bird out of the sky, and turns to the pathologist and says, "Go get it and tell me what it is."

A final poke at the three types of specialists.

What's the difference between an internist, a surgeon, and a pathologist? An internist knows everything but does nothing; a surgeon knows nothing but does everything; and a pathologist knows everything and does everything, but it's too late.

For better or worse, the perceptions of surgeons as "men" of action with big egos have solid historical origins. My surgical forefathers were bold, dynamic, egotistical, and almost universally male. Big egos were virtually essential to overcome frequent defeat and failure, and to continue the search for superior techniques and improved outcomes. I grew up with mantras like, "If in doubt, cut it out," and "A chance to cut is a chance to cure." As a surgical trainee who spent every other night on-call in the hospital looking after surgical emergencies, I was taught to complain that, "I'm missing half the cases!" Tough. Resilient. Tireless. These were the qualities that were valued, modeled, and rewarded.

Boy, what a hotshot!

Tough. Resilient. Tireless. I appreciate these qualities. But all of us involved in medical education have come to understand that being up every other night does not create a receptive learner, a good spouse, or a good parent. Nor does fatigue promote good patient care.

Residency = No Outside Life

Speaking of being a good spouse and parent reminds me that at one point in my career I was the program director of the General Surgery residency program. One of my jobs was to participate in career night for medical students. Program directors from the various residency programs would talk to the students about their speciality. During the Q&A that followed, I would invariably be asked to comment on the demands of a life in surgery. Students would ask me to comment on family life and rates of divorce. I would initially give a serious and honest answer. Then I would explain that I was happily married to my first wife, and had two children, and that my children were 5 years apart. And the 5 years between them were my exhausting residency years, during which time I had no sex. Then, after a brief pause, I would add, "I wish I could say the same about my wife." It always got a laugh.

While my teachers were all men, many of my colleagues and almost half of the residents today are women. All of my teachers were white. Now, thankfully, my colleagues and residents represent the diversity of Canada, one of the most culturally and ethnically mixed countries in the world. I should point out that gender equity in both leadership positions and income have not nearly been reached, but we are moving in the right direction.

A strong ego is still desirable. Surgeons must have confidence in their training and in their continuing professional development. They must trust in their knowledge, judgment, and skills. They have to know that they are able to focus and remain disciplined, no matter the circumstances. They must be able to weather the storm of self-doubt that follows every complication. This is especially difficult in the early years of a surgical career when a surgeon's reservoir of successes is shallow.

That being said, bravado is ruinous and unacceptable. In my department, we refer patients to one another, we get second opinions, and we help one another in the operating room. The best outcome for the patient is all that matters.

Colorectal Surgeons, in particular, need pretty strong egos. We think we are the most long-suffering of all surgical specialists. No other group of surgeons toils in an environment populated by gazillions of deadly pathogens. The gut bacteria, way more of them in the colon, rectum, and anus than in any other part of the gastrointestinal tract, not only cause many of the diseases that we deal with, they threaten to complicate everything we do. They don't just threaten. No group of surgeons has to worry about or deal with more frequent complications, especially infections, than we do.

What's more, infections do not show up on the day of the operation or over the next 2 or 3 days. They usually show up a week or more later. That means after almost every operation, we are worrying for the next 2 weeks. So, we are basically worrying *all the time,* day and sleepless night. Every ring of the phone, every beep of the pager, every text message generates an unpleasant Pavlovian response.

When complications do arise after our operations, they are often dangerous, and may demand mature clinical judgment, thoughtful decision-making, multiple patient assessments at all hours, and sometimes re-operation. And to top it off, infections that arise from anastomoses, that is, putting bits of bowel back together, may be the result of technical failure.

Technical failure ... a euphemism. It means that the surgeon may not have put the bowel back together *perfectly,* resulting in separation of the anastomosis and leaking of bowel contents. Consequently, every failed anastomosis feels like our personal failure. Every anastomotic *leak* is a declaration that we're no damn good. Every anastomotic failure is a professional existential crisis.

How often does this leak business happen? The leak rate is about 5% (some operations a bit higher, some a bit lower), but that's not the point. Every post-operative hiccup makes us worry about a leak, so we are worrying a lot. Even with a leak rate of 5%, a busy surgeon who does ten anastomoses per month will be dealing with anastomotic failure every other month. A lot of stress. A lot of self-doubt.

MASTER AND APPRENTICE

Patients often ask me if I will be doing the operation myself. The question is asked because I work at a teaching hospital and am involved in the training of General and Colorectal Surgeons.

Patients want to know, in other words, whether it will be me or one of my *trainees* doing the operation. My trainees are residents and fellows, Surgeons-in-training who have graduated from medical school (usually 4 years) and may have several years of surgical experience under their belts. The residency in General Surgery is usually 5 years (not counting research experience) and the fellowship (residency in a subspecialty) is usually an additional 2 years.

I explain to my patients that my trainees will be involved in their operation, but that I will be there from start to finish, either personally doing the operation or guiding every step of the operation. Not all teaching faculty work this way. I didn't always work this way. I used to provide residents with some independence, at least for some parts of some operations. But my approach has changed over the years and I am now present from the initial *check-list* until the final dressing has been applied, if not longer.

The check-list is an important contribution to modern surgery. Credit goes to Dr. Atul Gawande, who reviews the principles and evidence in his 2009 book, *The Check-List Manifesto*. Patients will be gratified to learn that in hospitals around the world, before an operation can be started, the team of Nurses, Anesthetists, and Surgeons huddle to go through a check-list. We make introductions if needed, and we run through a series of checks to ensure that we have the right patient (pretty important), that we are going to proceed with the right operation, and that all of the appropriate pieces are in place, including personnel, positioning, and equipment. We review the patient's allergies and other medical problems. We ensure that pre-op medications like prophylactic antibiotics (to prevent infections) and prophylactic anti-coagulants (to prevent deep vein thrombosis – DVT or blood clots) have been given. We confirm whether the patient is going home, to the ward, or to the intensive care unit (ICU) following surgery. We check with the patient whether they would like us to call a family member or friend at the end of the operation.

I also do a check-list at the end of the operation before the patient is awakened from anesthesia. The Scrub Nurse and the Surgeons clasp hands and take a few seconds to review that the instrument, sponge, and needle counts are correct; that we did what we came to do; that we didn't forget to do any of the things we came to do; and that the appropriate intraoperative checks were done. I call it *the circle of love*. A little team-building and an opportunity for me to say thank you to the team. It's also

Are you going to do my operation?

a final check before anaesthesia is reversed and the patient heads to the post anaesthesia care unit (PACU). (I can surmise what was wrong with *recovery room*, but it has taken some time to get used to *PACU.*)

Teaching technical skills during your patients' operations is problematic for Surgeons. Patients are not in the operating room (OR) to be practised on, but trainees cannot acquire all the skills they need just by watching and assisting.

There is pressure on the surgical teaching faculty to provide independence. A faculty member's Teaching Effectiveness Scores, generated by the residents and fellows, are used for assigning academic points, and these points are used in deciding faculty promotion and salaries. My scores aren't bad, but residents often comment that I am not providing them with as much operating as they feel they need.

The truth is, however, residents are never operating as much as they want or need. The learning curve is very steep and very long – lifelong.

Simulation models, a concept stolen from the airline industry, have proven extremely useful in teaching residents how to operate, reducing practising on patients. Simulations can also be used to help experienced Surgeons acquire new skills and as assessment tools in certification examinations.

But no matter what, Surgeons-in-training have to eventually do some *real* operating in order to learn the craft. The skills cannot be acquired by watching, by cutting along dotted lines laid out by their teachers, or by practising on simulation models. The learning experience must involve setting the pace and direction of operations, deciding on the sequence of steps that will safely and efficiently achieve the goals of the operation, and then executing those steps. Ushering trainees through every part of every operation and then letting them loose on the public to operate by themselves is not good for patients – or for Surgeons.

Independent operative experience can be safely provided to residents by ensuring that there is appropriate back-up and that an environment exists in which seeking help is a sign of mature judgment, not a sign of weakness – an environment in which patient safety and excellent outcomes are pre-eminent. A measure of the

competence and acumen of Surgeons at all levels is their awareness of their own limitations and their willingness to ask for help.
Confidence is good. Humility is better.

Too much independence; not enough independence. It's a fine line.
I have seen and personally experienced the negative consequences
of both insufficient oversight and excessive supervision.

During my residency in the early 1980s, for instance, the on-call
staff Surgeon did not have to come to the hospital at night or on
the weekend for emergency operations. The senior resident, at the
discretion of the staff Surgeon and after a telephone review, could
book (schedule) and perform emergency operations without the staff
Surgeon on the premises. This was insufficient oversight and I am
not aware of any teaching hospital that still allows this.

These days, the staff Surgeon must book the case and be in the
hospital, but there is usually no requirement that they be present
in the OR. This outside-yet-nearby approach balances the goals of
appropriate training and error-free operations.

Still, even when independence has been provided during training, the transition from residency to autonomous practice can
feel like falling off a cliff. The fall is made less precipitous and the
landing is softened by finding a senior colleague to act as a mentor.
Unfortunately, some young Surgeons fail to find a mentor and they
fall fast and hit the ground hard.

Transition to practice is a vulnerable time for newly minted
Surgeons and this phase in the arc of professional development is
beginning to get the attention it deserves. Rather than leave mentorship of the brand-new Surgeon to chance, many departments
have developed formal programs to support Surgeons who have just
completed their residency or fellowship. Many young Surgeons are
associates for the first year or two, with the expectation that there
will be help, as well as supervision, before being taken on as an
independent practitioner.

I feel guilty about not giving more independence to the trainees,
but as I got older I found that I was less able to give up control of

the operation. I try to assuage my guilt through teaching, and by allowing residents to do some parts of some operations, under my supervision, but without dictating every step and defining every plane of dissection. I try to teach and model behaviours that I think will help residents become successful Surgeons. I try to emphasize the attitudes that are fundamental to complication-free surgery, in particular, *focus, discipline, and humility.*

Focus is key because every operation is a series of steps, and every step is important. A Surgeon must never lose focus, not for a second.

But knowing every step and maintaining focus aren't enough. A Surgeon must have the *discipline* to insist that every step is done right. Decision-fatigue is a real risk, and being aware of it and not permitting it to affect one's judgment is critical.

As for *humility,* this is not a virtue conventionally associated with Surgeons. But ego has little place in the OR. Surgeons must be confident in their decisions and abilities, but we must also never forget that operations are all about the patient and not at all about the Surgeon. Asking for help is a sign of wisdom. It is not weakness. When the going gets tough during an operation, I say out loud, "Marcus, you're not as good as you think you are." It's my cue that it's time to slow down, take a deep breath, re-calibrate, and, occasionally, ask for help – before disaster strikes, not after.

It remains a personal struggle to balance the goal of providing an error-free, complication-free, executed-to-perfection operation, with the goal of providing an illuminating educational experience for my residents and fellows. For the record, I am still in pursuit of the perfect operation. I have come close a few times.

Perfection is a fascinating concept for Surgeons. Almost every Surgeon is taught that *perfection is the enemy,* or *perfection is the enemy of good.* I don't like that lesson and I don't teach it. I think I get it. In the pursuit of *perfection* you can screw up what was a *perfectly good result.* But I worry that it sends a message to accept *good enough.* And good enough usually isn't.

I want my operations to be perfect and I strive for that every time. I think the critical concept is to avoid perfectionistic behaviour, the tendency to never be satisfied. I have worked with Surgeons like this. They torture themselves and can actually injure their patients.

Do Surgeons acknowledge their mistakes? Yes. In fact, we think we do it better than any other group of physicians. On a weekly basis, we subject our performance and our patients' outcomes to the scrutiny of our peers. Surgical groups (services) have meetings, called *rounds,* in which diagnostic errors, near-misses, complications, and deaths are reviewed. These used to be called Morbidity and Mortality (M&M) rounds but are now called Quality Assurance (QA) or Quality Improvement (QI) rounds.

In the good old days, Surgeons, especially residents, used to be targeted by other members of the service and asked to defend their decision-making. Things could get ugly.

Modern QA rounds, unlike the M&Ms of the past, are not about pointing fingers and laying blame. Instead, the process seeks to identify aspects of patient management that could have been better. Sometimes improvement is needed at a system level, sometimes at the level of individual knowledge and skills.

Peer review is an essential element of surgical practice and it is deeply implanted in the surgical psyche. I fully embrace it. In the clinic, in the OR, in my interactions with colleagues, co-workers and trainees, I try to conduct myself in a way that would be assessed favourably by my peers if reviewed at the next QA meeting.

WHY I DO WHAT I DO

Sphincter-preserving operations attracted me to the Colorectal Surgery subspecialty, but why Surgery in the first place?

My answer has probably been shaped by the passage of time. I am not certain what my 24-year-old self was thinking when I applied to the General Surgery Residency Program. As an intern on the General Surgery service, I found that I admired the Surgeons.

And I liked the idea of being a Surgeon – not very sophisticated or altruistic thinking. I think I also wanted to be challenged and thought that Surgery would challenge me. I had no idea how true that was. More than 40 years later, I still find myself intellectually, emotionally, and, ever more, physically challenged.

Do I enjoy what I do?

I've had a love/hate relationship with my surgical career.

I have read that career satisfaction is primarily related to the degree to which three goals are achieved: meaning, mastery, and autonomy. This has stuck with me because I think it's true.

> *Career satisfaction is primarily related to the degree to which three goals are achieved: meaning, mastery, and autonomy.*

Meaning is pretty easy for doctors. Medicine is a service industry and the service we provide has value for our customers. We have the opportunity to make lives better and to save lives. It can feel pretty damn good and very meaningful. It can also feel rotten when things go wrong. None of us get through our careers without errors, some of which do harm to patients. Few of us get through our careers without bad outcomes, unhappy patients, complaints to a disciplinary body, or even a malpractice lawsuit. Still, the good we do dramatically exceeds the harm. I have a strong sense that the work I do is meaningful.

Mastery is also a pretty achievable goal for Surgeons, although it is less achievable than you might think. Personally, I was well into my career before my sense of mastery was well established. Even now I regularly question my judgment. And I always tread cautiously. Surgical decision-making and operative execution are mine fields. One wrong step ... kaboom. Each step needs careful consideration. Despite a strong sense of mastery, I remain very aware of my ability to make a mistake and I try to keep my wits about me at all times. Every second.

Lack of *autonomy* has been my greatest frustration. Surgeons in public health care systems have little control in their professional life. This often shocks patients. How much operating time is made available, how many cases can be scheduled, the order of the cases, access to the endoscopy unit, how often one is on-call, the number and level of the residents assigned, the experience and quality of the Nurses and OR technicians, access to ward beds, to intensive care unit (ICU) beds, to emergency OR time, how much one is paid for procedures, and one's teaching assignments – none of this is within the control of the surgeon.

Time in the OR is such a limited resource that there is tremendous pressure on Surgeons not to run late, not past 3:30 p.m. at many institutions.

Running late can easily happen. It is not usually because the Surgeon over-booked their operative list, or misjudged the degree of difficulty of an operation. These can certainly occur, but it is more often for reasons that were not within the Surgeon's control, like a post anaesthesia care unit (PACU) that's backed up, or an induction of anesthesia or awakening from anesthesia that took longer than expected, or a delay in the preparation of the room, or getting bumped by an emergency. When a case is running late, whatever the reason, it is the Surgeon who is required to cancel the next patient's operation. Administrators don't deal with the upset patient.

Once upon a time, Surgeons operated until the list of patients who had been scheduled was completed. Those days are gone and that's a problem. Ask yourself, "Would I rather be the last patient on the list or the next to last patient?" The last patient might get bumped. The next-to-last patient might have a Surgeon who is rushing so that they will not be forced to cancel their last patient. The threat of cancellation is not good for Surgeons or patients, but it is a reality in an over-burdened system. Most of us book our operative lists very responsibly, accepting that we will sometimes finish early. We focus on the quality of the operation in progress, looking away from the clock on the wall. We try.

Surgeons book cautiously, but there is a lot of pressure on us to fill our allotted OR time. There are long wait lists in publicly funded systems, and wasted OR time leaves patients lingering even longer. Hospitals do nothing to reduce the pressure on Surgeons. The opposite is true. I have attended meetings where OR administrators have talked about taking away OR time from Surgeons who finish early, since "they clearly have more time than they need." I have attended meetings where OR administrators have talked about taking away OR time from Surgeons who finish late, since "there need to be consequences for overbooking."

A lack of autonomy is closely related to the current state of most public health care systems. In these systems, Surgeons are not a resource centre, rather they are a cost centre. The more operations performed, the more it costs the system. For most of my career I have worked at about 75% of my personal capacity because of lack of resources, such as hospital beds and OR time. I have had wait times for elective surgery of over 2 years but it is hard to turn away patients, especially when it is unclear that they have somewhere else to go. All of my colleagues are in the same boat. I don't know a single Surgeon without a long wait list.

More patients than resources. Long wait lists. This creates what has been called moral injury for doctors working in a system of limited resources. Most Surgeons have some degree of moral injury resulting from the endless struggle to get their patients looked after. Trying to arrange the care for your patients generates more burn-out than does the care itself.

Despite these criticisms of a public health care system, I am an ardent supporter of the concept. It is a privilege to work in a system in which my patients do not have to pay me for their care, in which they do not have to calculate whether they can afford the care I am recommending, where they might have to choose a medically inferior option because it costs less, or might have to forego care altogether because they could not afford it.

I work at an inner-city, tertiary-care, trauma centre and teaching hospital. Homeless shelters, the stock exchange, the big banks, and law firms are right next door. As a result, the waiting room for my clinic has bankers and lawyers sitting next to people with no fixed address. They all are going to get the same level of care. And that care will invariably be associated with waiting. Being triaged to the top of the wait list is common in my practice, and it is based on the nature of the pathology, not on an ability to pay. That would give rise to a moral injury of an entirely different magnitude.

Meaning, mastery, autonomy. Meatloaf was right, *two out of three ain't bad.*

I remind myself how lucky I am to love my work, even if I don't love it all the time. Loving your work is a great gift. I sometimes feel like I have never really worked a day in my life.

Appendix

TOP TEN TIPS FOR ANAL HEALTH

1. Keep stool soft by eating a fibre-rich diet.

2. Drink fluids to stay hydrated.

3. Be physically active.

4. Don't ignore the call. If you gotta go, go.

5. Don't read, text, or email on the toilet.

6. Elevate your knees by resting your feet on something to approximate a squat position.

7. Don't strain more than a few seconds.

8. Wash and wipe gently.

9. Don't put anything up there that might get stuck.

10. Don't be afraid or embarrassed to see a doctor if you have concerns.

Glossary

abscess: A collection of pus within the body. [pages 37-40, 54, 57-59, 114-115]

adalimumab: Marketed as Humira®, it is an antibody that suppresses TNF (tumor necrosis factor), which is part of the inflammatory process. It is used in UC, CD and rheumatoid arthritis. [pages 108, 115]

adenoma/adenomatous polyp: A benign growth arising from the lining (mucosa) of the gut. [pages 23-24]

Altemeier procedure: Also called *perineal proctosigmoidectomy*, it is an operation for rectal prolapse in which the prolapsing segment is removed (resected) and the colon is anastomosed to the anus. It is an operation *from below* (from the perineal aspect). There is no abdominal incision. [page 67]

anal canal: The anal canal, or anus, is the terminal part of the GI tract. It begins at the anorectal junction and ends at the anal verge. The anal canal is surrounded by the internal and external anal sphincters. The lining of the anal canal varies depending on the location within the canal. The lining above the dentate line is the same lining as in the colon and rectum, called *columnar mucosa*. Below the dentate line is the anoderm, skin without sweat glands and hair follicles. Over 5-10 mm above the dentate line there is a transition zone with both types of lining. [pages 10, 12, 14, 29, 36, 54, 58, 79, 89-90, 135, 137]

anal fissure: A crack or tear in the anoderm. [pages 12, 14, 30-36, 43, 54, 100, 115, 130, 134, 135]

anal manometry: A test that measures pressures in the anal canal at rest and with squeezing. During anal manometry, the RAIR (rectoanal inhibitory reflex), rectal sensation, and the ability to expel a balloon from the rectum are also usually assessed. [pages 102, 103]

anal margin: The 5 cm zone around the opening to the anus. [pages 33, 89-90]

anal polishing: Excessive washing and scrubbing of the anus. It is also called *polished anus syndrome* and it is an important causative factor in primary pruritus ani. [pages 18, 48]

anal sphincter muscles: The internal and external sphincter muscles form the wall of the anus. The internal anal sphincter (IAS) is smooth muscle. It is a continuation of the circular muscle of the rectal wall. Smooth muscle is involuntary muscle (not under our control) and the IAS is responsible for resting anal pressure. The external anal sphincter (EAS) is skeletal muscle. It is voluntary muscle (under our control) and is responsible for squeeze pressure. [pages 20, 31, 34, 42, 78]

anal squamous cell carcinoma (A-SCC): The most common type of cancer arising from the anal canal and anal verge. The main cause is HPV (human papilloma virus). It is most often treated by a combination of chemotherapy and radiotherapy. Cure rates are related to the stage, but overall are 80% or higher. [page 89-90]

anal stenosis: An abnormal narrowing of the anus producing difficulty in the evacuation of stool. It can occur in Crohn's disease and as a complication of hemorrhoidectomy. [pages 21, 114]

anal verge: Where the anoderm meets the skin of the buttocks. [pages 11, 36, 135]

anastomosis: A surgical connection made between tubular structures. [pages 25, 103, 104, 111, 112, 117-118, 149, 154]

anastomotic leak/dehiscence: The partial or complete disruption or separation of an anastomosis. [pages 117-118]

anismus: Failure of relaxation of the pelvic floor muscles during the defecation effort. Because the muscles do not relax, the anorectal angle does not open, and evacuation is obstructed (obstructive defecation syndrome). [page 123]

anoderm: The lining of the anus below the dentate line. The skin of the anoderm differs from the skin of the anal margin in not having hair follicles or sweat glands. Where the anoderm meets the skin of the anal margin is the anal verge. Where the anoderm meets the lining (mucosa) of the upper anus is the dentate line. [pages 29, 30, 86]

anogenital: Relating to the zone around the anus and genitals. [pages 86, 87]

anorectal: Relating to the anus and rectum. [pages 4-6, 70, 72, 148]

anorectal angle: The angle between the anus and the rectum formed by the levator muscles. At rest, the angle is roughly 90 degrees. During evacuation, the levator muscles relax, the anorectal angle opens (becomes less acute), and the rectum empties. [pages 102, 103, 123-124]

anorectal junction: The transition from the rectum above the pelvic floor to the anal canal below is called the anorectal junction. The junction is where the rectum narrows as it passes through the pelvic floor muscles (levators), becoming the anal canal (anus).

anovaginal fistula (AVF): An abnormal connection between the anus and vagina. AVF is most often caused by trauma during vaginal delivery. [pages 70-75]

anterior: Toward the front of the body. [pages 30, 39, 58]

anterior resection: An abdominal operation in which part of the rectum is removed (resected) and an anastomosis is made between the colon and the remaining rectum. [pages 81-82]

anterior resection syndrome (ARS): The disturbance in bowel function that results from anterior resection, including frequency of bowel movements, nocturnal bowel movements, difficult evacuation of stool, and fecal incontinence. [pages 81-82]

anti-coagulant: Medication used to slow down the coagulation of blood; also called a *blood-thinner*. [page 155]

ARS: anterior resection syndrome

A-SCC: anal squamous cell carcinoma

ascending colon: The right colon, from the cecum (below the ileocecal valve) to the hepatic flexure (where the ascending colon meets the transverse colon). [pages 1, 26]

ASCRS: American Society of Colon and Rectal Surgeons [page 6]

autoimmune diseases: Diseases in which our immune system attacks part of our own body. [pages 108, 109, 112]

AVF: anovaginal fistula

balloon expulsion test: A test of defecation in which a balloon is inflated in the rectum, filled with 50cc of fluid, and then evacuated. Patients with obstructed defecation syndrome (ODS) have difficulty evacuating the balloon. This test is usually done as part of *anal manometry*. [pages 102, 103]

bile: A fluid secreted by the liver. Bile flows via a duct system (the bile ducts) into the duodenum (the first part of the small intestine) where substances in the bile aid in digestion. Pigments in the bile are responsible for the typical brown colour of stool. [page 125]

BM: bowel movement

Botox™: Botulinum toxin is a medication injected to decrease muscle contraction. [pages 33, 42]

bowel prep (preparation): A clean out of the bowel by laxatives (prep solutions) in preparation for colonoscopy and for some colorectal operations. [pages 17, 72, 139]

calcium channel blocker: A medication that inhibits muscle contraction. [page 32]

carcinoma: Cancer arising from the lining of internal organs like the intestine. [pages 23, 89]

CD: Crohn's disease

CD4: CD4 cells are T cells (a type of white blood cell) that are an essential part of the human immune system. [page 85]

cellulitis: Inflammation of the subcutaneous tissue. [page 40]

CI: colonic inertia

cloaca: A common canal for the vagina and the anorectum. A cloaca is a normal part of human embryonic development, before the vagina and anorectum become separate structures. Trauma to the region, especially obstetrical trauma, can produce a *traumatic cloaca.* [pages 70-71]

colitis: Inflammation of the colon. [pages 15, 108-113, 114, 148]

colon: The large bowel. [page 1]

colonic inertia (CI): *See* slow transit constipation.

colonic muscle wall: Over most of its length, the wall of the gut is formed by two layers of smooth (involuntary) muscle. An inner muscle coat has muscle fibres that are oriented in a circular pattern, and an outer muscle coat has longitudinally oriented muscle fibres. The muscles are responsible for the contractions and peristalsis that moves gut content from one end to the other. [pages 24, 31]

colonoscope: *(n)* A flexible fiberoptic instrument, 160 cm in length, for examining the colon; *(v)* to pass the scope. [pages 15, 16, 100]

colonoscopy: Examination of the colon with a colonoscope. [pages 15-17, 22, 23, 32, 66, 99, 113, 135, 138-142]

colon transit test: A radiologic test to measure the rate of transit of orally ingested markers through the colon. Patients with normal transit will have evacuated 20 radio-opaque (seen on plain x-ray) markers within 5 days. [page 102]

colostomy: A colonic stoma. The colon is brought out of the abdomen through an aperture in the abdominal wall and feces drain into a bag. [pages 71, 115, 116-118, 148]

colo-vaginal fistula: An abnormal connection between the colon and vagina. Colo-vaginal fistula is most often caused by sigmoid diverticulitis in patients who have had a hysterectomy (removal of the uterus). [page 26]

colovesical fistula: An abnormal connection between the colon and urinary bladder. Colovesical fistula is most often caused by sigmoid diverticulitis. It is the most common type of fistula to result form sigmoid diverticulitis. [page 25]

condyloma (condyloma accuminata): Anal warts. [pages 86, 88]

continence: The ability to defer the passage of stool, gas, or urine. [pages 20, 32, 33-35, 55-61, 65-66, 67, 70-75, 77-84, 111, 113, 115, 130]

Crohn's disease (CD): An inflammatory disease of uncertain cause that can affect any part of the gut. The inflammation may involve all the layers of the bowel wall. Inflammation may cause obstruction or perforation of the bowel. The inflammation can also affect other parts of the body, including the skin, joints, and eyes (so-called *extra-intestinal manifestations*). [pages 15, 54, 108-110, 113-115]

deep vein thrombosis (DVT): A blood clot in a vein. [page 155]

defecation: The discharge of stool (feces) from the body. [pages 30, 100, 101, 102, 103-104, 121-125]

defecation postural modification device (DMPD): A fancy name for a footstool, it was developed to replicate the alignment achieved with squatting during defecation. [page 124]

defecogram: *See* defecography

defecography (defecogram): Defecography (a poop-o-gram) is a radiological imaging examination in which the mechanics of defecation are visualized. The anatomy and function of the anorectum and pelvic floor are dynamically evaluated. It can be done with x-rays or with MRI. [pages 102-103]

Delorme: A perineal (from below) operation for rectal prolapse in which the rectal wall is plicated (corrugated or folded). [page 67]

dentate line: A wavy (tooth-like) line in approximately the middle of the anal canal where the lining of the upper anus (mucosa) meets the specialized skin (anoderm) of the lower anus. [pages 11, 12, 21, 38]

diverticulitis: Inflammation of a diverticulum. [pages 24-26]

diverticulosis: The presence of diverticula. [pages 24-26]

diverticulum: *(pl. diverticula)* An out-pouching (or sac) from the wall of a hollow organ like the colon. [pages 24, 26]

DPMD: defecation postural modification device

DVT: deep vein thrombosis

dyssynergic defecation: Failure of the pelvic floor muscles to relax during defecation efforts. It is the most common cause of ODS (obstructive defecation syndrome). [pages 103-104, 123, 127]

EAAF: endoanal advancement flap (*See also* Flap/endoanal advancement flap.)

EAS: external anal sphincter

endoanal advancement flap (EAAF): A "sphincter-preserving" operation for anovaginal fistula and other complex anal fistulas. (*See also* flap/endoanal advancement flap.) [pages 60, 72, 73]

endoscope: A flexible fiberoptic instrument for looking into body parts (e.g., gastroscope and colonoscope). [page 5]

enterostomal therapy/therapist (ET): A subspecialty of nursing focusing on the care of ileostomies and colostomies. Many ETs also have expertise in the management of complex wounds. [pages 116-117]

epidural anesthesia: A type of anesthesia in which the anesthetic agent is paced in the epidural space around the spinal cord. This is a type of *regional anesthesia.* [page 27]

episiotomy: A cut made at the opening of the vagina during vaginal delivery. [page 69]

ET: enterostomal therapy/therapist

EUA: examination under anesthesia

examination under anesthesia (EUA): An examination of the anus in the operating room under regional or general anesthesia, often done as part of the management of anal fistula, or to examine the anus in patients with painful anal pathology. [pages 41, 58, 59]

excise/excision: To cut out; the act of surgical removal. [pages 20, 37, 88, 90-91] external anal sphincter (EAS): The voluntary skeletal muscle forming the outer wall of the anus. [pages 11, 34, 38, 79]

fecal immunochemical test (FIT): The FIT is a screening test for colon cancer. It finds blood in the stool, which can be an early sign of cancer. It is the main alternative to colonoscopy for colon cancer screening. FIT is usually done annually or every two years. [pages 141-142]

fecal incontinence (FI): Lack of voluntary control over the passage of stool; inability to defer the evacuation of stool; *unwanted escapes; inability to get to the toilet in time to avoid an accident.* (The term fecal incontinence may also be applied to flatus incontinence, the inability to prevent the escape of gas.) [pages 65-66, 67, 70-75, 77-84, 130]

fecaluria: Stool in the urine. This is a symptom of a fistula between the GI tract and the urinary tract, most often between the sigmoid colon and the bladder resulting from sigmoid diverticulitis. [page 25]

feces *(adj. fecal):* The waste discharged from the bowel. [page 125]

fellow: A senior trainee (resident) in a surgical or medical subspecialty residency (training) program. A *fellow* has already completed a residency in a surgical or medical general specialty (like General Surgery or Internal Medicine) and is pursuing additional training and certification in a subspecialty (like Colorectal Surgery or Cardiology). [page 154]

Fellowship: A surgical or medical subspecialty training program, usually of 2 or more years' duration. [pages 47, 154]

FI: fecal incontinence

fissure: A crack or tear in the anoderm. [pages 12, 14, 30-36, 51, 54, 100, 115, 130, 134, 135]

fistula: An abnormal tunnel-like connection between two surfaces (e.g., between the anal glands and the skin around the anus). [pages 25, 39-40, 53-61, 114-115]

fistulotomy: An operation to treat an anal fistula in which the fistula is unroofed (laid open). [pages 55-58, 60, 114]

FIT: fecal immunochemical test

flap/endoanal advancement flap (EAAF): An operation for complex anal fistula (like an anovaginal fistula) in which a flap of anorectal tissue is developed and used to patch over the anal opening of the fistula. [pages 60, 72, 73]

flatus: Gas, fart. [pages 33, 35, 125-127]

GA: general anesthesia

gastrocolic reflex: Increased contraction of the colon in response to food or liquid entering the stomach. [pages 122, 133]

gastrointestinal tract: The tubular gut, from mouth to anus, plus the organs that secrete or carry fluids into the gut – the salivary glands, liver, gall bladder, bile ducts and pancreas. [pages 1, 3, 24, 25, 71, 108, 109, 150, 153]

general anesthesia (GA): Anaesthesia that affects the whole body, and includes loss of consciousness. [pages 27, 66, 88, 96]

GI: gastrointestinal (*See also* gastrointestinal tract.) [pages 99, 118]

gonococcal proctitis: Inflammation of the rectum due to gonorrhea. [page 85]

gracilis interposition: An operation for complex anal fistulas, like a large anovaginal fistula, in which the gracilis muscle is transposed from the thigh and interposed between the anus and the vagina, thereby interrupting (closing) the fistula. [page 74]

hemorrhoid: Internal hemorrhoids are normal structures located above the dentate line in the anal canal. They are thickenings of the anal lining filled with small blood vessels. These "vascular cushions" may protrude from the anus and may bleed. There are usually three cushions, often located in the left lateral, right anterior, and right posterior positions. External hemorrhoids are skin tags at the anal verge and may be associated with prolapsing internal hemorrhoids or may be independent problems. Unlike internal hemorrhoids, external hemorrhoids are not normal structures. [pages 7, 9-23, 38, 49, 51, 78, 82, 115, 124, 130, 134, 135-138]

hemorrhoidectomy: Excision of hemorrhoids. [pages 13, 17, 20-22, 115, 136-138]

hemostasis: Stopping bleeding. [page 61]

high resolution anoscopy (HRA): Enhanced inspection of the anus with a magnifying scope, used to identify and treat HPV lesions. [page 88]

HPV: human papilloma virus

HRA: high resolution anoscopy

human papilloma virus (HPV): A sexually transmitted infection associated with anal warts (condyloma accuminata), and with pre-cancer and cancer of the anus and cervix. [pages 51, 86, 87-89, 91, 129-130]

hypertonicity: Sustained and abnormally intense contraction of a muscle. [pages 31, 32, 34, 130]

hypertrophied anal papilla: Papillae (folds of tissue at the dentate line) may enlarge, especially in association with chronic anal fissure. It is also called a *fibrous anal polyp.* [page 31]

I&D: incision and drainage

IAS: internal anal sphincter

iatrogenic disease: Disease caused by the physician. [page 60]

IBD: inflammatory bowel disease

IBS: irritable bowel syndrome

ID: infectious disease (a subspecialty of internal medicine) [page 86]

idiopathic disease: A disease of uncertain cause. [page 108]

ileal pouch: A reservoir (pouch or neo-rectum) made from the ileum (last part of the small intestine). It is part of the operation called *ileal pouch anal anastomosis*, an operation used mainly in ulcerative colitis. (*See also* J-pouch and neo-rectum.) [page 111]

ileal pouch anal anastomosis (IPAA): An operation in which the colon and rectum are removed and an ileal pouch (reservoir) is anastomosed (attached) to the anus. It is most commonly done for ulcerative colitis. [pages 111, 112-113, 118, 148, 149]

ileostomy: An ileal stoma. The ileum (last part of the small intestine) is brought out of the abdomen through an aperture in the abdominal wall and ileal content drains into a bag. [pages 71, 74, 111, 112, 116, 148]

ileum: The last part of the small bowel. [pages 1, 71, 112, 148]

imiquimod: A medication for HPV (human papilloma infection). [page 88]

immunosuppressives: Drugs (medications) that suppress the immune response. An example is Imuran™, a trade name for azathioprine. [page 108]

incision and drainage (I&D): An operative incision that allows an abscess to drain. [pages 40, 54]

inflammatory bowel disease (IBD): A group of diseases associated with inflammation of the colon and small intestine. Ulcerative colitis affects the rectum and part or all of the colon. Crohn's disease can affect any part of GI tract, including the small intestine, the large intestine, the mouth, the esophagus, the stomach, and the anus. [pages 15, 81, 107-120, 149]

infliximab: A medication, brand name Remicade®, used to reduce inflammation. It is an antibody mainly used to treat autoimmune diseases, such as IBD. It is administered by intra-venous infusion at 6-8-week intervals. [pages 107, 108, 115]

internal anal sphincter (IAS): The ring of smooth (involuntary) muscle that surrounds the anal canal. The IAS is responsible for approximately 80% of the pressure within the anal canal (resting anal pressure). The IAS transiently relaxes as gas or stool enter the rectum (sampling reflex). The IAS is one of the critical mechanisms in providing continence for stool and gas. [pages 31, 32, 34, 57, 79, 103, 130]

intra-colonic pressure: The pressure within the colonic lumen. [page 24]

intussusception: In-folding of the wall of a tubular organ. Rectal prolapse is an intussusception of the rectum. [pages 64, 103, 104]

IPAA: ileal pouch anal anastomosis

irreducible: Not able to be reduced. This term is often used in the context of a prolapsing hemorrhoid or a rectal prolapse in which the prolapsed tissue is *stuck* in a prolapsed position. [page 13]

irritable bowel syndrome (IBS): A disease of gut function with a wide range of symptoms, including abdominal pain, bloating, diarrhea, constipation, and irregularity. Anxiety, depression, and chronic fatigue syndrome may be associated with IBS. [pages 18, 81, 100]

J pouch: A pouch (reservoir) surgically constructed from adjacent limbs of bowel to function as a "neo-rectum." A J-pouch may be constructed from the terminal ~40 cm of the ileum in the IPAA operation. A J-pouch may also be made from the colon and anastomosed to the anus or lower rectum following rectal resection. (*See also* ileal pouch and neo-rectum.) [pages 111-112]

keyhole deformity: An abnormal notch or groove at the anal verge. It may result from anal surgery but is mainly a risk from fissurectomy (which is no longer done for chronic anal fissure). [page 35]

laparoscopy: An operative method where scopes and instruments are inserted into the abdomen through small incisions in the abdominal wall; also called *MIS* (minimally invasive surgery). [page 66]

laparotomy: An operative incision that enters the abdominal cavity. [page 94]

lateral: Toward the side. [page 35]

lateral internal sphincterotomy (LIS): An operation for chronic anal fissure in which some of the internal sphincter muscle is divided, reducing anal tone and improving anodermal blood flow. More than 90% of chronic anal fissures heal following LIS; there is a small risk of diminished continence associated with LIS. [pages 33, 34-36, 115]

left colon: The colonic segment from the region of the splenic flexure to the top of the rectum. The left colon comprises the descending colon and sigmoid colon. [page 12]

lesion: A site of damage to tissue through injury or disease. [pages 22, 40-41, 80, 90, 99, 100, 135, 139]

levator muscles: A group of muscles, also called *levator ani*, that make up the floor of the pelvis. The levator muscles, especially the puborectalis part of the levators, create the anorectal angle, an important part of the fecal continence mechanism. The levators must relax during the defecation process and their failure to relax is a cause of ODS (obstructive defecation syndrome). The levator muscles contract when we cough or sneeze to prevent the escape of content from the rectum and the bladder. [pages 38, 41, 42, 123]

LI: loop ileostomy

LIFT: ligation of the intersphincteric fistula tract

ligation of the intersphincteric fistula tract (LIFT): A sphincter-preserving operation for complex anal fistula. [page 60]

LIS: lateral internal sphincterotomy

loop ileostomy (LI): An LI is most commonly made at the time of a rectal or anal anastomosis to divert stool away from the anastomosis during the early post-operative period. In this context, the LI is usually closed about 12 weeks later. An LI may also be made to divert stool from downstream disease, like severe anal Crohn's disease. [pages 117-118]

loperamide: A medication that slows muscle contractions (peristalsis) in the gut. It is mainly used to treat diarrhea and can be helpful in the treatment of patients with fecal incontinence. [pages 82-83]

lumen: The central cavity or channel of a hollow or tubular organ like the colon or rectum. [pages 23, 26]

magnetic resonance imaging (MRI): An imaging technique to examine parts of the body. [pages 41, 60, 90, 102]

manual reduction: Using the fingers to push back in tissue protruding from the anus, like hemorrhoids or rectal prolapse. [pages 13, 136, 137]

metastasize: The spread of cancer (malignancy) from the site of origin to a distant site, such as lymph nodes or other organs, like the liver and lung. [page 23]

minimally invasive surgery (MIS): An operative method where scopes are inserted through small incisions. Also called *laparoscopy*. [page 66]

MIS: minimally invasive surgery

motility: Movement. In the case of gut motility, it refers to contractions of the muscular wall of the bowel. [pages 82, 101]

MRI: magnetic resonance imaging

mucosa: The lining of the bowel. [pages 12, 14, 23, 24, 70, 72, 109]

multiparous woman: A woman who has given birth more than once. [page 64]

neo-rectum: A reservoir made out of small intestine or colon to replace the rectum after it has been resected (removed). (*See also* ileal pouch and J pouch.) [page 111]

neo-vagina: A vagina that is surgically created, usually as part of gender affirmation surgery. [page 74]

neurotransmitter: A substance released from a stimulated nerve that travels across a gap (synapse) to stimulate muscle or another nerve. [page 32]

nitroglycerine (NTG): A chemical used in medicine to relax smooth muscle like the internal anal sphincter in patients with chronic anal fissure. Its use can be limited by the side-effect of headache. [page 32]

non-relaxing puborectalis (NRPR): A common cause of ODS (obstructive defecation syndrome), it is a failure of the puborectalis to relax during defecation, thereby preventing the opening of the anorectal angle and blocking the exit of rectal contents. In a variation of NRPR, called *paradoxical puborectalis*, the puborectalis muscle contracts during evacuation efforts, making the anorectal angle smaller and evacuation impossible. NRPR is also called *anismus, dyssynergic defecation,* and *spastic pelvic floor.* [page 123]

NTG: nitroglycerine

nulliparous woman: A woman who has not given birth. [page 64]

obstructive defecation syndrome (ODS): Inability to easily evacuate rectal content leading to long periods of sitting on the toilet, manual manoeuvres to aid in evacuation, straining, and ineffective evacuation. [pages 101-104]

ODS: obstructive (or obstructed) defecation syndrome

overlapping sphincteroplasty: An operative technique to reconstruct disrupted anal sphincters. [pages 73-74, 83]

paradoxical puborectalis: *See* non-relaxing puborectalis.

pathology: The study of the causes and effects of diseases. The branch of medicine that deals with the examination of samples of body tissue for diagnosis. [pages 4, 16, 23, 39, 41, 47, 51, 56, 66, 121, 136, 142]

patulous anus: An anus with little or no tone or squeeze. [page 65]

PEG: polyethylene glycol

pelvic floor: The muscles that form the base of the pelvis. [pages 20-21, 38, 41-42, 64-65, 67, 80, 82, 83-84, 98, 101, 103-104, 105, 123-124]

perianal: A non-specific term referring to the region around the anus. [pages 18, 22, 32, 51, 88, 89, 90, 129, 145]

perineal proctosigmoidectomy: An operation for rectal prolapse in which the prolapsing segment of rectum and colon is resected. The non-prolapsing colon is anastomosed to the anus. The operation is done from below (perineal approach). It is also called the Altemeier procedure. [page 67]

perineum: The region between the anus and the scrotum or vulva. [pages 70, 73]

Pico-Salax®: A type of laxative. [pages 97, 101]

pneumaturia: Gas in the urine. It is almost always the result of a fistula between the GI tract and the bladder. The most common fistula to the bladder is from the colon due to sigmoid diverticulitis. [page 25]

podophyllin: An ointment for anal warts. [page 88]

polyethylene glycol (PEG): A type of laxative often used for bowel preparation. [pages 32, 101]

polyp: A non-specific term for a protrusion into the lumen of a hollow organ. The most important polyps of the GI tract, called *adenomas,* arise from the mucosa of the colon and rectum. Adenomas are important because of their potential to become malignant. This is the polyp-cancer (adenoma-carcinoma) sequence. [pages 15, 16, 17, 22, 23-24, 81, 136, 139-142]

pouchitis: Inflammation of an ileal pouch (reservoir). [pages 112, 113, 119]

prednisone: A steroid medication to reduce inflammation. [page 107]

proctoscope: An instrument with a light for examining the anus and rectum. [page 5]

proctoscopy: Examining the anus and rectum with a scope. [pages 15, 75]

prolapse: Displacement of an organ from its normal position in the body resulting in it protruding from an orifice. [pages 12, 13, 63-68, 81, 130, 135, 137]

pruritus ani: Anal itch. [pages 18, 43, 45-52, 89]

psyllium: A plant, the seeds of which are used as a dietary fibre supplement (bulking agent) to help regulate bowel function. [pages 31, 82]

RBL: rubber band ligation

rectal prolapse: Intussusception of the rectum in which the lead point of the intussusception extends through the anus to the outside. [pages 63-68, 130]

rectoanal inhibitory reflex: A relaxation reflex of the internal anal sphincter (IAS) in response to rectal distension. The reflex is tested as part of *anal manometry*, a series of tests that measure pressure and sensation in the anus and rectum. Distension of a balloon in the rectum causes the IAS to relax with a resultant drop in the resting anal pressure. Absence of the reflex is seen in a congenital condition called Hirschsprung's disease in which there is an abnormality of the nerves of the rectum. [page 103]

rectopexy: An abdominal operation for rectal prolapse in which the rectum is anchored to the sacrum, either by sutures or by prosthetic mesh material. [page 66]

rectus abdominis muscles: The "six-pack" muscles of the abdominal wall. [page 117]

reduce: To manually push back in protruding tissue, like grade III hemorrhoids or a prolapsing rectum. [page 13]

regional anesthesia: A technique to take away sensation in a part of the body, like epidural anaesthesia often used in obstetrical care. [page 36]

resect: To remove a section of the bowel. Resection can be restorative (the bowel is put back together with an anastomosis) or non-restorative (an ileostomy or colostomy is established). [pages 25, 26, 81-82, 99, 110, 114, 148] residency: A period of specialized training in a field of medicine. [pages 152, 154, 157]

resident: A medical school graduate (doctor) training in a field of medicine. [pages 56, 152, 154, 156-159]

RP: rectal prolapse

rubber band ligation (RBL): An office treatment for internal hemorrhoids in which tight elastic bands are applied to the hemorrhoids. Also called *banding*, it is a common treatment for grade II and small grade III internal hemorrhoids, but not used for external hemorrhoids (skin tags). [pages 17, 19-20, 137]

sacral nerve stimulation (SNS): A procedure for fecal and/or urinary incontinence in which an implanted pacemaker stimulates the nerves to the pelvic floor muscles (the sacral nerves), including the anal sphincter and the urinary bladder. [pages 83-84]

sacral neuro-modulation: Another name for the sacral nerve stimulation (SNS) procedure. [pages 83-84]

sampling reflex: The reflex relaxation of the internal anal sphincter that occurs when material enters the rectum. The reflex allows rectal content to enter the upper anus where specialized nerves send signals telling us whether the material is solid, liquid, or gas. [page 79]

seton: A strand of material used in a fistula operation. [pages 58-60, 115]

sigmoid colon: The part of the colon just above the rectum. [pages 24-25, 71]

sigmoid diverticula: Diverticula in the sigmoid colon. [page 24]

sigmoid resection: Resection of the sigmoid segment of colon. [page 25]

SIL: squamous intraepithelial lesion

skin tag: A prominent fold of skin at the anal verge. [pages 14, 37, 78, 110, 137]

slow transit constipation: Constipation that is due to the slow movement of stool through the colon. Also called *colonic inertia*. [pages 100, 101-104]

SNS: sacral nerve stimulation

somatic nerves: Highly sensitive nerves in the body wall. [page 12]

spastic pelvic floor: Failure of relaxation of the pelvic floor muscles during the defecation effort; because the muscles do not relax, the anorectal angle does not open, and evacuation is obstructed (obstructive defecation syndrome). [page 123]

sphincter disruption: A tear in the sphincter. [pages 72, 74, 80, 83]

sphincteroplasty: Operative repair of the sphincter. [pages 73-74, 83-84]

spinal: *See* epidural anaesthesia.

squamous intraepithelial lesion (SIL): A pre-cancerous change in the anoderm secondary to HPV infection. [pages 88, 89, 91]

STC-IRA: subtotal colectomy with ileorectal anastomosis

stenosis: Narrowing of a channel, such as the anus, rectum, or colon. [pages 21, 113, 114, 137]

steroids: A family of compounds that can be used to dampen the inflammatory response. [page 108]

STI: sexually transmitted infection. *See* human papilloma virus.

stoma: A surgically made opening on the body that leads into a hollow organ. Ileostomy and colostomy are types of stomas. [pages 71, 73, 116-118, 148]

stomal hernia: Enlargement of the opening (aperture) made for a stoma in the body. [page 117]

stricture: An abnormal narrowing (stenosis) of a hollow organ like the colon. Colonic strictures can be benign (e.g., due to inflammation) or malignant (e.g., due to colon cancer). [pages 25, 26, 99]

subtotal colectomy with ileorectal anastomosis (STC-IRA): A restorative resection in which the entire colon is removed and the small bowel is attached (anastomosed) to the rectum. [page 103]

TEH: thrombosed external hemorrhoid

terminal ileum (TI): The last segment of small bowel that joins the large bowel. [pages 113, 139]

thrombosed external hemorrhoid (TEH): A tense, tender, purplish, painful lump at the anal verge. It may result from a tear in a vein, thrombosis (clotting) in a vein, or a combination of these. It may occur spontaneously, but often results from straining at stool or heavy lifting. [pages 36-37, 38, 39, 135]

TI: terminal ileum

TNM: tumor, node, metastasis

tubular adenoma: A type of benign growth arising from the lining (mucosa) of the gut. Adenomas have the potential to become carcinomas (cancers). [page 23]

tumor, node, metastasis (TNM): A staging system for cancer that refers to the extent of the disease, such as how large the tumor (T) is and whether or not it has spread (metastasized) to lymph nodes (N) or distant organs (M) like the liver or lungs. [page 90]

UC: ulcerative colitis

UI: urinary incontinence

ulcer: A break in the mucosa (or the skin) that fails to heal. [pages 30, 43, 90, 134]

ulcerative colitis (UC): An idiopathic (of uncertain cause) inflammation of the rectum and a variable amount of colon. In UC, unlike Crohn's disease, the inflammation does not affect the anus or the small bowel. [pages 15, 49, 108-120,148, 149]

unroof: Lay open. [pages 55, 57, 114]

urinary incontinence (UI): Unwanted escape of urine. [pages 80, 83]

ventral mesh rectopexy: An abdominal operation for rectal prolapse in which a mesh is placed along the front (ventral) wall of the rectum to prevent intussusception of the rectal wall. [pages 104-105]

visceral nerves: Nerves that run to and from the internal organs. Unlike somatic nerves, which provide very discrete information about heat, cold, and pain, the visceral nerves provide duller sensations. This is why, for example, polyps can be removed from the colorectal lining (polypectomy) and internal hemorrhoids can be tied off (rubber band ligation) without pain. [page 12]

.

About the Author

Marcus J. Burnstein, MD, MSc, FRCSC, is an Associate Professor of Surgery at the University of Toronto. Dr. Burnstein trained in General and in Colorectal Surgery at the University of Toronto and in Colorectal Surgery at the Lahey Clinic Medical Centre in Massachusetts. He is a past program director for the University of Toronto Residency Programs in Colorectal and General Surgery, past chairman of the Royal College Specialty Committee for Colorectal Surgery, and past president of the Canadian Society of Colon and Rectal Surgeons.

A former member of the Board of Directors of the American Board of Colon and Rectal Surgery, Dr. Burnstein continues to serve as a senior examiner for the Board. He is an associate editor of the *Canadian Journal of Surgery* and has been an associate editor for *Diseases of the Colon & Rectum.*

Dr. Burnstein has a broad practice in diseases of the colon, rectum, and anus at St. Michael's Hospital in Toronto.

www.ingramcontent.com/pod-product-compliance
Lightning Source LLC
Chambersburg PA
CBHW051723020426

42333CB00014B/1118

9 781738 109302